Stress and Coping in
Mental Health Nursing

Stress and Coping in Mental Health Nursing

Edited by

J. Carson

Lecturer in Clinical Psychology, Institute of Psychiatry, London, UK

L. Fagin

Consultant Psychiatrist, Forest Healthcare Trust, London, UK

S.A. Ritter

Lecturer in Psychiatric Nursing, Institute of Psychiatry, London, UK

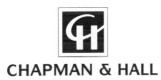

CHAPMAN & HALL

London · Glasgow · Weinheim · New York · Tokyo · Melbourne · Madras

**Published by Chapman & Hall, 2–6 Boundary Row,
London SE1 8HN, UK**

Chapman & Hall, 2–6 Boundary Row, London SE1 8HN, UK

Blackie Academic & Professional, Wester Cleddens Road,
Bishopbriggs, Glasgow G64 2NZ, UK

Chapman & Hall GmbH, Pappelallee 3, 69469 Weinheim, Germany

Chapman & Hall USA, One Penn Plaza, 41st Floor, New York
NY 10119, USA

Chapman & Hall Japan, ITP-Japan, Kyowa Building, 3F, 2-2-1
Hirakawacho, Chiyoda-ku, Tokyo 102, Japan

Chapman & Hall Australia, Thomas Nelson Australia, 102 Dodds
Street, South Melbourne, Victoria 3205, Australia

Chapman & Hall India, R. Seshadri, 32 Second Main Road, CIT East,
Madras 600 035, India

Distributed in the USA and Canada by Singular Publishing Group Inc.,
4284 41st Street, San Diego, California 92105

First edition 1995

© 1995 Chapman & Hall

Typeset in 10/12 Palatino by Mews Photosetting, Beckenham, Kent
Printed in Great Britain by Page Bros., Norwich, Norfolk

ISBN 0 412 59270 3   1 56593 330 3 (USA)

A catalogue record for this book is available from the British Library

Library of Congress Catalog Card Number: 94-68773

∞ Printed on permanent acid-free text paper, manufactured in
accordance with ANSI/NISO Z39.48-1992 and ANSI/NISO Z39.48-1984
(Permanence of Paper).

Contents

Contributors

Heather Bartlett
Community Psychiatric Nurse, Thornbury Day Care Unit, London, England

Daniel Brown
Psychologist, Institute of Psychiatry, London, England

Philip Burnard
Senior Lecturer, Cardiff, Wales

Tony Butterworth
Professor of Community Nursing, School of Nursing Studies, Manchester, England

Jerome Carson
Lecturer in Clinical Psychology, London, England

Lynda Dunn
Psychologist, Institute of Psychiatry, London, England

Leonard Fagin
Consultant Psychiatrist, Claybury Hospital, Woodford Green, England

Kevin Gournay
Professor of Mental Health, Middlesex University, Enfield, England

Jocelyn Handy
Senior Lecturer, Massey University, Palmerston North, New Zealand

John Leary
Clinical Psychologist, Claybury Hospital, Woodford Green, England

Peter Nolan
Lecturer in Nursing Studies, Medical School, University of Birmingham, England

Susan A. Ritter
Lecturer in Psychiatric Nursing, Institute of Psychiatry, London, England

David Rushforth
Lecturer in Nursing, School of Nursing Studies, Manchester, England

Roisin Stewart
Research Worker, University of Ulster, Belfast, Northern Ireland

Barry Tolchard
Nurse Behaviour Therapist, Guy's Hospital, London, England

Foreword

Philip Burnard

Mental health nursing, like the whole of the profession, is undergoing rapid change. Change always involves stress – few people cope very well with stress and those in the mental health field are particularly vulnerable. This is true from both consumer and carer points of view. The health care consumer is having to face radical governmental changes in policy. The carer faces the prospect of the mental health nursing qualification being changed out of all recognition. Carers and consumers will have to learn to cope in order to survive.

All of this occurs in an even larger context of change – that of the national picture of health care. Students and practitioners in the mental health care field will be aware – on an almost daily basis – of the cuts and redevelopments of almost all aspects of the national health care system in the UK. This can be demoralizing or exciting, depending on your particular position in the organizational hierarchy and on your beliefs about how health care should be delivered. Either way, it is another contributor to stress in the profession. One thing seems certain: the rate of change may vary in the next few years but the **fact** of change will not alter. Any of us working in the health care professions can expect that considerable change is yet to come.

This book is a welcome and timely addition to the literature. It offers an overview of the history of mental health care, it places it in context and offers a range of studies into stress in mental health nursing. While there are many books about individuals coping with stress, this one is different in that it offers descriptions, analyses and prescriptions. It is not a simple 'how to get rid of stress' book but an important and accessible view of all aspects of stress in the mental health nursing profession. As the first of its kind, it will be welcomed by students, educators and clinical practitioners. The editors are to be congratulated in bringing together key figures in the profession to write chapters for this volume. The editors' contributions are also of paramount importance in helping the reader to contextualize and make sense of the other writers' work.

Stress and Coping in Mental Health is important from a number of points of view. First, it will supply background information about the mental health nursing profession that is not available elsewhere. Second, it offers the reader two things from the point of view of research: it offers the findings of various studies into stress; it also offers the methodologies that were used to complete these research projects. This sort of information will be essential reading for the student who is new to the field or for the researcher who wants to develop his or her own work. The book also has direct relevance for those at the sharp end of the mental health field – the practitioners who are working with clients in hospitals and in the community. The book constantly highlights the political and cultural aspects of stress and coping – issues that are often left out of books on stress. Too often, stress is viewed as being something 'personal', experienced by the individual in an apparent social vacuum. This book offers a clear view of the whole of the mental health nursing field – historical, political, social and personal. It will be essential reading for anyone who has anything to do with health care provision.

Dr Philip Burnard
University of Wales College of Medicine, Cardiff

CHAPTER 1

The development of mental health nursing

Peter Nolan

INTRODUCTION

There are many reasons why members of a profession should want to examine their own history. Being part of a group with a long tradition of service to society confers respectability and legitimizes one's work, promoting a sense of civic pride. It is important to know the circumstances in which a particular profession came into existence because the words and deeds of its founding fathers (or mothers) often become a template for the work of their followers and act as a yardstick against which to measure, in future decades, how far the profession has evolved or deviated from its original philosophy.

Those who set out to examine the history of mental health nursing must confront the fact that there has never existed, and still does not exist, a unique philosophy of mental health nursing which structures its practice. Nor is there any substantial body of historical data about mental health nursing to which reference can be made, such as that accumulated by the Royal Colleges of Surgeons, Physicians or Psychiatrists. Instead, what we have are snapshot accounts of institutional care at different times and in different places, records written at the whim of certain literate nurses and preserved by chance.

This chapter is based on the assumption that the origins of modern mental health nursing can be found in the asylum system because it was within the asylums that nursing took shape, evolving pragmatically, shaped by outside influences such as that of the Medical Superintendents and the members of the Boards of Governors of the asylums. Until very recently, nurses themselves have had very little influence over what has happened to their practice and their profession, although a minority have tried hard.

Prior to 1845, the year in which the Lunacy Act made statutory the building of specialist institutions, many mentally ill people were incarcerated either in workhouses or in prisons where their needs went unrecognized. Some care was available in the private sector, but this tended to be generally poor in quality. Madhouse owners exercised control over disturbed patients by means of leg irons, straitjackets and starvation, rather than by employing extra staff. They tended to take far too many patients in order to maximize profits. Conditions in these houses were appalling as we know from William Tuke, founder of the Retreat, who described the plight of his niece, 'cared for' at the York Asylum. Unwashed, she lay on straw soiled with her own faeces, semistarved and so dehydrated that she tried to drink her own urine (Digby, 1985).

It would be wrong, however, to point only to poor practices in the 18th and 19th centuries when there were also notable examples of humane care. Doctors such as Thomas Bakewell and Nathaniel Cotton ran excellent, well-respected establishments where many patients made full recoveries (Smith, 1992; Nolan 1990). Both these men believed that the success of their regimes depended largely on those they employed as 'servants' to the residents. Through the servants, the care and understanding that are the hallmark of a civilized society were transmitted to its suffering citizens. All the servants had their own residents to attend to (a precursor of the 'named nurse' system); discussion amongst staff about the care to be given took place every morning and the day was punctuated by gatherings of residents and servants to read the Bible, listen to music or take walks in the country.

THE CREATION OF THE ASYLUM SYSTEM

The man who most ardently pleaded for the creation of a specialist system to look after the mentally ill was the great humanitarian reformer, Lord Shaftesbury. Shaftesbury had been convinced by eminent doctors such as John Connolly that mental illness was in essence like any other type of illness and simply needed greater investigation for cures to become available. He therefore argued in Parliament that a system of institutional care for the insane would provide opportunities for patients to be studied scientifically and treatments tested with the ultimate aim of eradicating mental illness. During the debates initiated by Shaftesbury, all aspects of the proposed institutional life were discussed, with the notable exception of who was going to care for the patients on a day-to-day basis, and how. An atmosphere of therapeutic optimism prevailed when the first asylums were built in 1845 and there is no doubt that the asylum system regulated the haphazard provision of care previously available, but the new system was founded on no carefully considered ideas about practical care.

The new institutions were almost immediately overwhelmed by large numbers of people from the workhouses, many with chronic physical as well as mental conditions. Within a short period, over 90% of asylum inmates were classified as paupers (Korman and Glennerster, 1990). Overcrowding was inevitable because the asylums were expected to be self-financing and Medical Superintendents aimed to generate income by admitting as many patients as possible, particularly people from outside the asylum's catchment area for whom considerably more was paid than the standard rate for patients from within the locality. The Committee of Visitors at the Lancaster Asylum reported in 1852 that:

> At the commencement of the year 1851, there were in the asylum 785 patients, a number far too great for the comfort and well-being of the inmates; and such has been the pressure for accommodation that every available space was obliged to be used.

As there was no money to provide for extensions, the only recommendation contained in the Report was that the cemetery should be enlarged!

The attendants employed to look after the mentally ill occupied the middle ground between doctors and patients. Socially and intellectually, their status was far inferior to that of the medical staff, but their closeness to the patients made them highly influential in the day-to-day running of the asylums. For the most part, more was expected of the attendants than their background and lack of training made it possible for them to deliver. The financial pressure placed on the asylums meant that Medical Superintendents aimed to employ attendants who could provide all the skills required to run their institutions. The Worcester County Asylum appears to have been very successful in achieving this:

> Most of the attendants are artisans who work with patients, do all the repairs and anything requiring attention. The shoemaker takes chief charge of the First Convalescent Ward as well as overseeing the shoe-repair shop. The mason takes charge of the Second Convalescent Ward: he is glazier, painter and decorator. The tailor assists in the Fourth or Epileptic Ward at meal-times and in the evenings. The Fifth Ward has two attendants: the junior takes charge of the barrow-men and assists in all excavations and wheeling of earth. It is only by such arrangements that any asylum can be conducted efficiently.
> *(1851 Annual Report of the Worcester County Asylum)*

Male attendants were commonly regarded as the 'unemployable of other professions' and, socially, the stigma of the insane rubbed off on them (Carpenter, 1980). In the majority of asylums from the 1850s to the late 1890s, no training was provided for attendants, and no effort was made to define their duties and help them understand what they were expected to do. Life for the attendants was hard and dangerous. Appalling incidents took place such as the case outlined in the 1860 Annual Report of the Prestwich Asylum:

> One of the oldest attendants, John Tetlow (remarkable for his habitual kindness to those under his charge), was stabbed most severely in the mouth by one of the patients. The wounds, which were extremely dangerous in character, were inflicted by means of a dinner knife. The knife passed through the cheek and deeply penetrated the root of the tongue, causing a fearful haemorrhage ... However, he did recover and to his credit, be it said, he remains an attendant still ... The patient ... was irritated during dinner time by another patient purloining his bread and struck at him in consequence with his knife. Two of the attendants went to his rescue and Tetlow received his injuries in the struggle.

The Report concluded that, regrettably, there would be occasions when attendants would be the subject of serious assaults, but that this was no reason for curtailing the liberties and comforts of the patients.

The personal diary of Mr Newman, an attendant at the Wiltshire County Asylum in Devizes (latterly called Roundway Hospital), contains fascinating details about the attendants (Nolan, 1993). Some were referred to as 'solid' or 'stout men'. Their background was in farm labour and they were cherished by Superintendents because they could contribute to the running of the asylum farm and therefore to the income of the institution. Because they were physically strong, they could also help to administer unpleasant treatments of the type generally regarded by patients as punishments. To subject someone to the 'bath of surprise', cold showers or the swivel chair took a considerable amount of strength. Keeping these particular attendants proved difficult because they were easily tempted away to more lucrative agricultural work, especially during the summer months.

Another group of workers comprised members of families in which institutional work was carried on from one generation to the next. Superintendents learned to ask those whom they considered good employees whether they had children or relatives who might be interested in working at the asylum. The children of staff benefited from having realistic expectations about the work of an attendant and from the supervision and advice of their parents.

Newman goes on to describe the type of attendants who had previously been in service to the gentry as butlers, footmen, gardeners or labourers. These men were used to taking orders and to working long hours for little pay. A small group of male attendants comprised ex-servicemen from the army and navy who were much liked by

Superintendents because of their disciplined background and their ability to lead and be led.

The majority of asylums followed the general hospitals in referring to female carers as 'nurses'. Nurses were drawn mainly from those who would otherwise have gone into domestic service. The attraction of asylum nursing lay in the full board and lodgings it provided, but the work was harder than service to the gentry and the only social life to which the women could look forward was going home on their days off or meeting, at infrequent intervals, some of the male attendants. Male and female attendants were required to remain in their own areas of the asylum and mixed only rarely on sporting and social occasions when their communications had to be discreet. In the event of marriage, the women lost their posts. Older women who went into the asylums were generally widows and were preferred by Superintendents because they were already accustomed to hard work and did not complain about conditions of service. No particular skills were required of them other than being able to cope with long hours and hard work.

Long hours of duty meant that attendants were exposed without respite to often highly disturbed patients and had to cope as best they might with the kind of violent incident described above. The stresses involved in caring for the mentally ill did not go unrecognized within the asylums and were made more tolerable for staff by the provision of facilities for sport, especially football and cricket. Sporting activities became a key feature of asylum life, fulfilling the dual purpose of keeping attendants fit and so able to deal with the attacks they encountered on the wards and offering them an acceptable way of venting their own frustrations and aggression. By the turn of the century, the facilities for sport provided by most asylums were instrumental in attracting many people to work there.

TRAINING FOR THE ATTENDANTS

The limited training available for attendants during the first 50 years of the asylum system was matched only by the poverty of training available to doctors. Apart from the *Journal of Mental Science*, there were few opportunities for doctors to learn about the latest theories of mental illness and new treatments. Although certain individuals tried to improve the state of specialist psychiatric knowledge – Alexander Morrison, Inspector of Asylums, started inhouse lectures for doctors at the Bethlem Hospital in 1823, John Connolly at the Hanwell Asylum in 1842 and Thomas Laycock in Edinburgh in the 1860s – it was not until 1885 that the Medico-Psychological Association (MPA) persuaded the General Medical Council to introduce a Certificate in Psychological

Medicine. Prerequisites for the Certificate examination were that candidates should have been resident in a mental hospital for three months and attended a course of lectures. Nobody applied for the first examination (Lewis, 1967).

Training for attendants had been started by doctors in various asylums, but it was unregulated and patchy. In 1885, the MPA attempted to address this situation by commissioning a training manual to help standardize the various courses for attendants running up and down the country. *The Handbook for the Instruction of Attendants on the Insane* contained 64 pages, was bound in red hardboard and had an appendix that listed all the public and private asylums in the UK and their Superintendents. It proclaimed that the first duty of attendants was to impose discipline on patients by setting an example of industry, order, cleanliness and obedience. The text was divided into chapters under the following headings:

1. The body: its general functions and disorders
2. The nursing of the sick
3. Mind and its disorders
4. The care of the insane
5. The general duties of attendants.

The Handbook was a watershed in the history of mental nursing because it represented a shift from the oral tradition, through which the work of mental nurses had previously been described and handed on, to a written one.

In response to the attendants' manifest eagerness for knowledge, a second book appeared in 1886 entitled *Lectures on the Care and Treatment of the Insane, for the Instruction of Attendants and Nurses*. Written by Dr Williamson, Medical Officer for the Insane at Paramatta, the Introduction to the 70 page book states:

> No mere book-reading will make a good attendant out of bad one. Nevertheless, we believe that a few well-chosen practical directions will help to make a good attendant better.
>
> (Williamson, 1886)

Williamson considered the attendant's role was to carry out medical instructions while carefully supervising the patients. Supervision, he found, was often inadequate:

> Black eyes, cut faces, bruises and scalp wounds received by epileptics or by other patients in conflict with them are in a large number of instances evidence of lack of proper supervision.
>
> (Williamson, 1886)

Williamson's book was enlarged upon by Strachan (1886) who argued that the work of the attendants demanded a more rigorous training to encompass not only the elementary principles of nursing, but also consideration of how their work fitted into the broader medical context of psychiatry. Strachan felt that a greater understanding of mental illness would enable attendants to deliver treatments more effectively and hence improve the outcome for patients. Lobbying from Medical Superintendents, combined with the desire on the part of the attendants to learn as evidenced by their voluntary attendance at informal training courses, finally convinced the Medico-Psychological Association that a national training scheme was overdue. Its 1889 Annual General Meeting unanimously approved the appointment of a Special Committee to investigate the possibility of awarding a Certificate in Nursing the Insane and the registration of certificate holders.

The Committee decided on a three month probationary period to be served before attendants could be accepted for training. This was followed by 21 months of training and service in the asylum. The Handbook was ordained as the basic training text, but other books could be made available to trainees at the discretion of their Superintendent. Lectures and demonstrations were given by medical staff, although occasional practical exercises might be supervised by the Head Attendant. These lectures were usually held in the evenings for staff who had often been on duty since 6.00 am. In some asylums, probationers were expected to stand during lectures to prevent their falling asleep! The Superintendent assessed trainees' progress by periodic tests.

Examinations were held twice yearly on the first Monday in May and the First Monday in November in each asylum where there were candidates. The examination fee of 2s 6d had to be paid by the attendant at least four weeks before the examination date; resits were charged at 1s. There was both a written paper and a *viva voce* with questions being set by the same members of the MPA who examined medical students for the Association's Diploma. Written answers were marked by the attendants' own Superintendent and also by an outside assessor who was usually a Superintendent from another asylum approved by the MPA to act in this capacity, with the *viva voce* being conducted by the same two Superintendents.

The introduction of training did not, of course, change the situation within the asylums overnight. Staff who had been selected following the briefest of interviews and who had subsequently received only the most superficial training could not be expected to behave like well-educated, professional people. In an extensive study of attendants in the West Midlands during the 19th century, Smith (1988) found that doctors had expectations of the attendants which their background and lack of education meant that they could not fulfil. The lunacy reformers and administrators realized that unsatisfactory nursing staff were adding to the problems in the asylums caused by severe over-crowding, but beyond the provision of basic training, the Medico-Psychological Association did not attempt to address the situation of either patients or attendants within the asylums. It provided no ongoing training for attendants and did not invite them to participate in the Association's meetings or to become members of its commit-tees. Attendants were excluded from all professional activities.

The medical profession found the introduction of training for the attendants a useful public relations exercise. To have trained nurses on the wards enabled doctors to argue that caring for the insane was skilled work and so helped them refute charges of inadequacy and amateurism arising out of psychiatry's lack of a theoretical framework or scientific knowledge base. The attendants gained little, if anything, from the new training scheme. After they had received their certifi-cates, they were not better off in terms of pay, conditions of service or career opportunities. There was no clear difference in status between the untrained attendant and the trained, a situation which did nothing to improve morale or standards of patient care. Moreover, trained attendants were liable to public humiliation and serious penalties if they failed to satisfy their Superintendents. Incidents of misconduct, ranging from petty theft, drunkenness and consorting with members of the opposite sex to assault on patients, all of which had been dealt with at local level prior to the advent of the Register, now entered the public domain.

UNINTENDED CONSEQUENCES OF TRAINING

Training did not diminish the tight control exercised by Superintendents over attendants, nor allow the attendants any greater independence of practice. The oppressive regime of the asylums made it difficult for attendants to form pressure groups and all attempts to unionize were fiercely opposed by Superintendents who dismissed anyone thought to be politically active. Determined to improve their working conditions, the attendants met at venues outside the asylums and one such meeting at the Boar's Head Hotel in Preston on the 24th September, 1909, saw the formation of the National Asylum Workers' Union (NAWU). Fuelled by resentment of the Superannuation Act (1909) which legislated for deductions towards a pension scheme to be made directly from attendant's wages, membership of the Union grew rapidly. Superintendents stubbornly refused to acknowledge the Union or to meet any representatives to discuss pay or conditions of service.

This attitude of the Superintendents combined with the harsh conditions endured by the attendants within the institutions led to the first strike in the history of mental health care on the 4th and 5th September, 1918. Three asylums were involved. At Prestwich Asylum, 200 staff came out; at Whittingham, 429, and at Winwick, a small number of attendants stopped work for a short period on both days. The following month, a five day strike was held at Bodmin Asylum where female employees tried to draw attention to their long hours of duty, bad working conditions and the systematic petty tyranny to which they were subjected. Nurses at Bodmin took to wearing their union badges openly whilst on duty, resulting in the Superintendent dismissing 50 of them. A Visiting Committee was quickly convened to hear evidence from the Superintendent and staff and decree that all the nurses who had been dismissed should be reinstated and allowed to wear their badges as long as these did not cause injury to patients.

More strikes took place during the early 1920s in Manchester, Lincoln and Nottingham and the NAWU took credit for exposing the harsh treatment of both patients and staff. The Union presented its charter for reform to Neville Chamberlain in 1923 which included:

- Improved quality of training;
- Shorter on-duty hours;
- Measures to reduce the rapid turnover of staff;
- Wages increased to the level of pay enjoyed by those in similar work outside the asylums;
- Measures to protect staff from infectious diseases;
- Review of the anomalies in the Asylum Officers' Superannuation Act 1909

MENTAL HEALTH NURSING BETWEEN THE WARS

The First World War won for psychiatry public recognition and appreciation and, as a result of it, the standing of psychiatry was greatly improved. Psychiatrists were deemed to have made a significant contribution to the war effort by treating thousands of men suffering from shell-shock and returning them 'cured' to the battlefield. Riding high on the nation's victory, psychiatrists saw the first psychiatric teaching hospital in Britain, the Maudsley, opened in 1924 and in 1926 were further rewarded when the MPA became the Royal Medico-Psychological Association. Also in 1926, Craig and Beaton's *Psychological Medicine* (Craig and Beaton, 1926) reached its fourth edition, consolidating a limited knowledge base with its classification and symptomatology of medical disorders and in 1927, the first edition of Henderson and Gillespie's *A Textbook of Psychiatry* (Henderson and Gillespie, 1927) appeared.

The mental hygiene movement also took root at this time. Its aim was to limit the incidence of mental illness by a programme of prevention which would start before birth. Pregnant women were to be advised about diet, exercise and infection risks so that they might provide the best possible environment for their developing babies. Such creative thinking and the changes taking place in psychiatry found no parallel within mental nursing which was still being practised as it had been for the previous 40 years. The *Journal of the National Asylum Workers* was more interested in portraying nurses as working class heroes; overworked, dedicated and lowly paid, than in addressing issues of practice and progress. By contrast, the *Nursing Mirror* (1922) was quite clear about the need for reform in mental nursing and considered it should move immediately in the direction of becoming more like general nursing.

There were indeed moves afoot to bring mental nursing into line with other areas of nursing. The Nurses' Registration Act for England, Scotland, Wales and Ireland received royal assent at the end of 1919 and the General Nursing Council (GNC) acquired authority to oversee the training of nurses and to draw up codes of practice and maintain standards. It introduced its own training for mental nurses which was very similar to that run by the Medico-Psychological Association and set up a Register for general nurses with a supplementary section for mental nurses. In May 1920, the General Nursing Council agreed that holders of the MPA's Certificate and those holding the recently established Certificate for Nurses in Mental Subnormality should be eligible for admission to its supplementary Registers. The first cohort of mental nurse trainees sat the GNC's examination in 1922. Of the 161 nurses who passed, 113 were female. The numbers of mental nurses registering with the GNC rose steadily until 1930 and thereafter, approximately 5000 nurses were registered annually, of whom an increasingly large percentage were women. The GNC's and the MPA's training courses ran side by side from 1922 until 1951, a situation which tended to promote confusion and division amongst mental nurses with some hospitals favouring MPA trained nurses and others GNC, although it was mostly MPA trained nurses who got promotion.

While the GNC was in the early stages of manoeuvring to bring all nurses under its aegis, psychiatry and mental nursing took a blow from the publication of Montagu Lomax's *Experiences of an Asylum Doctor* (1922). Based on his experiences as a doctor at Prestwich Asylum in Manchester, Lomax undertook a thorough indictment of the asylum system from which no-one escaped blamefree. Superintendents were accused of laziness, vanity and lack of management skills; nurses were sympathized with for their poor working conditions and the boredom of their daily routine, but castigated as a group largely uncaring and unimaginative in their approach to patients. Lomax exposed the poor food which patients received in the asylums, the poor clothing they were forced to wear and the appallingly mindless regimes to which they were subjected. The book was profoundly influential and resulted in a Royal Commission to investigate conditions in the asylums and, more significantly, a further enquiry, conducted independently of the MPA, to look at mental nursing.

The latter enquiry published its Report in 1924 (*Report of the Committee on the Administration of Public Mental Hospitals*, 1992) and presented conflicting evidence which on the one hand pointed to the unique nature of mental nursing and on the other, suggested that mental nursing should base itself on general nursing and its training format. The Report also failed to give a clear lead on whether the GNC should take control of mental nursing. Its overall effect was to confuse mental nurses as to whether their work was a branch of general nursing or a profession entirely separate from it.

The Report was stronger in those sections which recognized that in order for improvements in patient care to take place, there must first be improvements in working conditions. It therefore aimed to enhance the environment of the asylums by providing social facilities and academic opportunities for staff. Hospitals were urged to set up a nurses' infirmary and ensure a separate bedroom for each nurse and a private nurses' sitting room and dining room. At this time, the younger staff often slept in the patients' dormitories; nor did they have access to their own sitting room to which they could retreat in their time off. It is not surprising, therefore, that staff ran the wards for their own convenience and that pilfering of food and other items intended for patients was rife. The Report suggested that staff accommodation should be in a different building so that staff could receive their visitors without having to take them through the hospital. It urged management to provide more sporting facilities and indoor recreation in the form of dances, concerts, whist drives and billiards.

With reference to training, the Report recommended that teaching should take place in purpose-built schools of nursing, suitable for fostering the corporate life of students. Ideally, the schools were to be separate from the hospitals and set within their own gardens. The initial period of tuition for nursing students was to be free from ward duties.

The Report embodied a laudable attempt to improve the social lives of staff and give them an opportunity to escape the hospital routine and its isolationist culture. Sadly, its recommendations were not acted upon because neither the economic climate nor the will of the Superintendents was behind it. The nurses themselves were not consulted as to the content of the Report and few even heard about it.

While progress in improving working conditions for mental nurses was thus stagnant, changes in psychiatry were afoot. Insulin and electroconvulsive therapies and forms of occupational therapy were being introduced by doctors, with some nurses taking on a new role as their assistants, thus bringing the medical and nursing professions closer together. This new working relationship was further reflected in uniform culture with male nurses starting to wear white coats like doctors and female nurses dressing more like their counterparts in the general hospitals. Nurses involved in medical treatment of patients were seen as, and saw themselves as, superior to those who continued the traditional tasks of supervising patients at work on the farm, in the gardens and in the workshops, helping to service the hospital. A division began to emerge between 'clinical' and 'supervisory nurses'. Those who became clinically orientated tended to undertake general training after completing their mental nurse training and were much more successful in the promotion stakes. Those who concentrated on caring for the patients felt that their unique skills as mental nurses were being devalued.

IMPACT OF THE SECOND WORLD WAR

In the early 1940s, many nurses were called up, including some who were still in training, and assigned to the Royal Army Medical Corps. There they learned to handle medical emergencies and acquired psychotherapeutic skills which they would not have covered in training. The Maudsley Hospital was overwhelmed with soldiers suffering from neurasthenia and conversion hysteria and in 1940, a boarding school was converted into the Mill Hill Emergency Military Hospital with Dr Maxwell Jones in charge. Jones was later to treat many ex-prisoners of war returning from Japan at the Henderson Hospital in Sutton. Nurses working at the Maudsley and at Mill Hill were involved in exciting new approaches to the care of very disturbed patients.

Psychiatric hospitals and wards all over the country were cleared of patients in order to accommodate the large numbers of soldiers with war-induced mental health problems. The subsequent overcrowding coupled with low staffing levels increased the barely contained discontent amongst mental nurses. Problems increased when, after the war, many staff returned from Mill Hill or from the front with skills beyond the scope of those who had stayed at home. Their new skills went singularly unrecognized with older staff who had been recruited in their absence, often from Ireland, receiving promotion over their heads. Dissatisfaction was made worse by the drafting in of nurse tutors from the general hospitals to teach nursing care. Mental nursing staff, and especially those who had seen service, felt humiliated when taught how to set up trays and trolleys for medical procedures by general nurse tutors whom they considered had nothing to teach them about the care and management of the mentally ill.

Conditions for nurses and the treatment of patients remained, on the whole, lamentable. It is clear that many staff were still working through the terrible experiences they had endured during their military service or as prisoners of war. Demobilized soldiers were attracted into mental nursing by the military-style atmosphere of the hospitals and the excellent sporting facilities. Many of them had little time for the patients whose depressions, obsessions and anxieties they considered petty since these people had contributed nothing to the war effort. A 'macho culture' existed amongst the male nurses, fed by war memories of violence and the humiliation of people by enforced control. Part of this culture was, inevitably, the physical abuse of patients (Nolan, 1987).

A male mental nurse who started his career in 1947 records his first impressions thus:

> I was given a cubicle at the end of a dormitory. When it was decided that I was useful, I was given a room. The last meal was at 4.00 pm; the lights were put out at 10 o'clock and we were up at 5.30 am. The Charge Nurses were in complete control of their wards and nobody ever challenged them. Many of them spoke in a bullying and threatening manner ... They were men who were familiar with violence from the war. I was a coward – I should have done something about what I saw, but those to whom I would have had to complain were part of the same system.
>
> (Nolan, 1993)

THE HOSPITAL ENQUIRIES

During the 1950s, some nurses finally began to wake up to the negative effects which the monotonous and authoritarian routines of the mental hospitals might have upon patients whose mental health was already compromised. Attempts were made to transform institutional life from within. Cameron and Laing (1955) reported the initiatives of nursing staff who set aside time to be with patients, for getting to know and understand them and helping them to understand themselves. The Chief Male Nurse at De La Pole Hospital in Yorkshire, Mr P. Archer, introduced weekend leave for patients and a support network for those discharged home and worked successfully with the Medical Superintendent, Dr Bickford, to achieve improvements in patient care. Such initiatives were patchy, however, and were overwhelmed by the scandalous hospital enquiries of the 1960s and 1970s which exposed overcrowding, understaffing, low morale and the widespread abuse of patients by mental nurses. Despite having been taken into the National Health Service in 1948, many of the mental hospitals had continued to provide care for patients along lines laid down during the early days of the asylum system in the mid-19th century. Nurses were found responsible for perpetuating regimes which were uncaring when not overtly cruel. They were accused of having no respect for patients and no understanding of what mental nursing entailed. Their training was exposed as inappropriate for the work they were expected to do on the wards. Public opinion was outraged and government committed itself to the abolition of institutional care for mentally ill people. Just over a century had elapsed since the opening of the first asylum under the 1845 Lunacy Act; now totally discredited, the era of widespread institutional care was coming to an end.

DEINSTITUTIONALIZATION AND ITS EFFECTS ON MENTAL HEALTH NURSING

Mental health nursing came into existence to serve the asylums and was shaped more by the needs of the institutions and those who managed them than by the needs of patients. In spite of hard work, antisocial hours and lack of training, nurses developed strong attachments to 'their' asylum because well into the 20th century, the mental hospitals were tightly knit communities made up of families and close relatives where nursing was handed down from one generation to the next. Marriages between members of staff were frequent and weddings were often conducted in the hospital chapels with the hospital chaplain, choir and organist in attendance. The majority of staff lived either in hospital accommodation within the grounds or in hospital houses close by and bought their fuel, vegetables and dairy produce from the institution at much better prices than could be obtained elsewhere.

Recreational activities were a central feature of mental hospital life. Weekly dances and concerts were important in the social life of staff, as were the big sporting occasions when all staff would turn out to support the hospital team at cricket, football or athletics. The culture of mental hospital nursing was a very 'cosy' one for those nurses who were well integrated and did not complain of the minor and major abuses of patients carried out on the wards. Jones (1979) has described how, as the asylums grew in size, their routines became ever more rigid and the institutionalization of staff and patients became ever more complete. The support network amongst nurses was all the tighter because of the distance kept by the Medical Superintendent, under whom and generally against whom staff organized to protect themselves. Although training was largely irrelevant to the work nurses were doing, this was not a problem while nurses taught each other what to do within a highly effective oral tradition that flourished behind the closed doors of the institutions.

The isolation of the mental hospitals which had fostered and protected the community nurses was breached when the old asylum system started to be disbanded. In the 1960s, many of the hospital farms were sold and patients no longer went out in groups supervised by nurses to work on the land or in the gardens and workshops. Chemotherapy, group and occupational therapy replaced the therapy of outside work. In the 1970s, hospital houses began to be sold off and staff were encouraged to seek their own accommodation rather than depending on the hospital to supply it for them. As the hospitals became less self-contained, sporting and social activities came to an end and a shift in staff attitudes occurred so that the hospital was no longer a focus of allegiance but merely a place in which to work. Staff now moved readily between hospitals and were not expected to remain at the hospital where they had trained. In previous decades, such movement had never been encouraged and, indeed, was very difficult because nurses' knowledge of nursing care was tied intimately to the traditions of the particular institution which they had first joined.

The flow of staff and patients into the community which began as a trickle in the 1960s after the hospital enquiries became a flood in the 1980s. The transformation in the care of people with mental health problems took place on a scale and at a speed quite unprecedented in the history of nursing (Barham, 1992). The rundown of the mental hospitals happened far faster than alternative services within the community could be set up. Staff, like patients, were bewildered and the transition for them, despite the training they received in community nursing, was alarming and stressful. Traditional nursing wisdom was irrelevant to caring for clients in their own homes or in hostels and the isolationist cult of the mental hospitals made establishing working relationships with social services, the voluntary sector and primary care teams a very strange experience for many staff displaced from the institutions.

Community care is a public activity, quite different from the asylum system which operated behind closed doors. In the community, nursing practice is on view for all to see and criticize; within the institutions, nurses worked in secrecy and were largely unchallenged. In the community, different people with specialist skills are caring for clients with mental health problems; channels of communication are far more complex than in hospitals. There are also more opportunities for innovative care than were possible within the institutions, but such opportunities bring with them their own stresses to those unused to independent thinking. Redundancy is a constant threat as health districts are forced to cut back their staff in order to acquire trust status.

As mental health nurses strive to implement the reforms of the late 1980s and early 1990s, they find themselves under increasing pressure to take on larger workloads and cope with more difficult clients. They are continually exposed to a wide range of people with varying problems, much more so than other professional groups who tend only to see clients with a specific problem and for a short period of time. New roles and new skills are needed if the individual needs of clients are to be met successfully. The type of training that was pre-eminent in the past, aptly described by Cormack and Fraser (1975) thus:

> Training produces nurses who have no specific therapeutic role and therefore are forced to work in a role defined by the prevailing ideological situation

will have to be abandoned and replaced by training which will enable nurses to become independent thinkers, confident to make their own decisions in assisting people in all the varied contexts of their lives. Caring for clients in the community also involves caring for and supporting the families and friends with whom they are living. The training which mental health nurses currently receive, reduced in most cases to an 18 month branch programme since the introduction of Project 2000, cannot equip them to cope with the problems they are now daily encountering. There are some within the nursing establishment who seek the abolition of all nursing specialities and propose instead the 'nurse for all occasions', the generic nurse. It is questionable whether a generalist training in counselling and communication skills can sufficiently prepare nurses to deal with the consequences of severe mental illness.

There is much that can be learned from the past. The asylum system was established as a result of discussion and was not founded on any concrete evidence that it would be effective. Once built, the institutions were left to finance themselves. It soon became apparent that the running of a cost effective service and the provision of high quality care were often incompatible. A similar situation prevails today when resources are being directed away from the mental hospitals, but not ploughed into the community where government expects professionals to deliver a cost efficient and client centred service. Mental health nurses are thus finding themselves unable to practise satisfactorily either in the community arena or in the hospitals. As resources are drawn away from the hospital sector, only the most severely mentally ill can be admitted so that acute admission wards, more than ever before, now contain extremely disturbed clients whose care is highly stressful for an ever-reducing number of nurses. Ironically, these conditions return nurses to their Victorian roles of mere supervision and containment.

Community care involves a challenge which will be ignored by nurses only to their own cost. It is a challenge which takes nurses beyond the traditional boundaries of their profession, as laid down in the institutions, into the arena of social policy and politics:

> The problem with community care is not just about management. It is about misery (and) poverty . . . The kind of service provided by mental health professionals is not only or necessarily even the main issue that determines the quality of people's lives in the community.
>
> (Beeforth *et al.*, 1990)

Change of whatever sort places people under stress, but also provides opportunities for those brave enough and sufficiently creative to seize them. Mental health nurses now have the chance, as never before, to make their mark on the services provided for clients with mental health problems. After a century and a half of practice, a literature of mental health nursing is beginning to emerge, developed by mental health nurses themselves. When the asylum system was set up, it was doctors who wrote about nursing and taught nurses what they were to do; at the end of the 20th century, nurses have the chance to reverse that situation and to research their own practice. If they are truly alert to the voice of the client, mental health nurses will be aware that, despite all its difficulties, clients prefer to be cared for at home or in the community than in hospital. Nurses, of all people, must respond to such feelings because, if they do not, society has a right to consider that the basis upon which their profession is established has been discarded.

REFERENCES

Annual Report of the Worcester Asylum (1851) Archives of Powick Hospital.
Annual Report of the Committee of Visitors at the Lancaster Asylum (1852) Lancashire Records Office, HWH 24.
Annual Report of the Prestwich Asylum (1860) Lancashire Records Office, HWH 24.
Barham, P. (1992) *Closing the Asylum*, Penguin Books, Harmondsworth.
Beeforth, M., Conlon, E., Field, V., Hoser, A. and Sayce, L. (eds) (1990) *Whose Service Is It Anyway?* Research and Development for Psychiatry, 134–8 Borough High Street, London SE1 1LB.
Cameron, J.L. and Laing, R.D. (1955) Effects of environmental change in the care of chronic schizophrenics. *Lancet*, 1 1384–6.
Carpenter, M. (1980) Asylum nursing before 1914: a chapter in the history

of labour, in *Rewriting Nursing History*, (ed. C. Davis), Croom Helm, London.

Cormack, D. and Fraser, D. (1975) The nurses' role in psychiatric institutions. *Nursing Times*, **17**(5) 125–7.

Craig, M. and Beaton, T. (1926) *Psychological Medicine*, J. & A. Churchill, London.

Digby, A. (1985) *Madness, Morality and Medicine – A Study of the York Retreat*, Cambridge University Press, Cambridge.

Henderson, D.K. and Gillespie, R.D. (1927) *A Textbook of Psychiatry*, Oxford University Press, Oxford.

Jones, K. (1979) Deinstitutionalisation in context. *Millbank Memorial Fund Quarterly/Health and Society*, **57**(4), 18–24.

Korman, N. and Glennerster, H. (1990) *Hospital Closure*, Open University Press, Milton Keynes.

Lewis, A. (1967) *The State of Psychiatry*, Routledge and Kegan Paul, London.

Lomax, M. (1922) *The Experiences of an Asylum Doctor*, George Allen & Unwin, London.

Nolan, P. (1987) Jack's story. *History of Nursing Bulletin*, **2**(2), 18–21.

Nolan, P. (1990) The servant, the poet and the doctor: an example of 18th century psychiatric care. *History of Nursing Journal*, **3**(2), 3–13.

Nolan, P. (1993) *A History of mental Health Nursing*, Chapman & Hall, London.

Report of the Committee on the Administration of Public Mental Hospitals; 1922, Cmd 1730 viii, 185.

Smith, L.L. (1988) Behind closed doors: lunatic asylum keepers 1800–1860. *Social History of Medicine*, **1**, 301–27.

Smith, L.L. (1992) To cure those afflicted with the disease of insanity: Thomas Bakewell and Spring Vale Asylum. *History of Psychiatry*, **4**(13), 107–28.

Strachan, S.A.K. (1886) Can the medical spirit be kept up in asylums for the insane? *Journal of Mental Science*, **32**, 349.

Williamson, M. (1886) *Lectures on the Care and Treatment of the Insane, for the Instruction of Attendants and Nurses*. Privately published.

CHAPTER 2

Issues in the development of community mental health nursing services

Tony Butterworth and David Rushforth

PRECIPITATING FORCES

It is interesting to consider the development of community mental health nursing services at a point some 34 years since the first reported service was described at Warlingham Park Hospital (May and Moore, 1963). At that time, although nurses had worked in an 'extramural' capacity for some years previous to this first description, it was the first documented report of psychiatric nurse activity in the community setting. The World Health Organization had offered some ways of redirecting psychiatric care towards the community. In a report in the middle of the 1950s (WHO, 1956) they described nurses working before and after the hospitalization of people with mental illness in order to:

1. provide emergency care in the patient's home;
2. visit regularly at home to prevent admission to hospital;
3. shorten lengths of stay in hospital by early discharge and continued visiting.

Hunter (1974) ascribed these tasks to the work of the various community psychiatric nurse services which were beginning to develop 15 years later but added practical tasks such as bathing and shaving and helping patients to find jobs and accommodation as the core work of community mental health nursing. He also emphasized the importance of the family and nurse relationship. Greene (1968), in describing the role of the mental health nurse, suggested that the activities of nurses could be summarized in the following way:

To provide psychiatric nursing care of a physical or psychological nature in accordance with the doctor's wishes for patients who have been discharged from hospital and who are in need of continuing nursing care ... working in close liaison with doctors and social workers as professional members of a therapeutic team ... extending to the patient and his family such support as may be reasonably regarded as part of nurses' work ... a preventive role in going to the aid of patients whose illness does not require treatment in a clinic or hospital ... being available in a con-sultative capacity to non-psychiatric nurses who may have problems with patients showing symptoms of nervous and mental disorders.

It is possible to recognize many of the characteristics of those early services as being present in today's community mental health nursing activities.

A number of small scale surveys had showed a steady growth in service provision such that by 1974 there was a fairly even spread of services nationally (Carr *et al.*, 1980). Their value and effectiveness were frequently reported but these changes in influence and practice were under-researched.

A sudden growth of service provision during the 1970s has been linked to the then new Local Authority Social Services Act which precipitated a new generic role for social workers and forced con-siderable changes on social service provision. Specialist psychiatric social workers became all but extinct with the advent of the 1970 Act. As contact with social workers by people with mental illness reduced there was considerable anecdotal evidence to suggest that nurses both exploited and filled the gap left by social workers and indeed were encouraged to do so by professional colleagues and service managers.

Numbers in the workforce have now reached approximately 5000 with a projected figure by 1995 of almost 7000 (White, 1990).

LOCATION OF SERVICES AND PATTERNS OF REFERRAL

There has been a tendency until recent times to consider services as working in teams and having an identifiable base. However, this simple approach is becoming more complicated by new services pro-vision under the reorganized health service. Location of service does have an effect on the nature and origin of referrals and the type of people nurses will see and work with. There is some weight to the belief that referrals from psychiatrists have a positive association with people who have a history of mental illness and hospital admis-sions, with chronic mental illness and with people who have a diagnosis of schizophrenia. Referrals from general practitioners have a negative correlation with these categories (White, 1990). It is also possible to say that nurses working from a hospital base receive more referrals from psychiatrists whereas nurses in non-hospital bases have a greater proportion of referrals from general practitioners and that nurses working from hospital bases have more clients on their case-loads who have serious and enduring mental illness and/or a diagnosis of schizophrenia and previous admission. It cannot be assumed that this implies a universal criticism of base location; indeed, if services offer referral systems which make them open and accessbile to psychiatrists then referrals from psychiatrists may be higher (Brooker and Simmons, 1985).

CASELOADS AND THEIR COMPOSITION

A number of surveys have been conducted which have examined the nature of the work of community mental health nurses. The most recent (White, 1990) gives a wealth of data about the work patterns and caseload of community mental health nurses. Data from this survey are used here to illustrate service developments. The mean caseload size for community mental health nurses in England in 1990 was 34.3 people. Proportions of these caseloads show those with a previous hospital admission (47.9%), those with chronic mental illness (42.6%) and those with a diagnosis of schizophrenia (26%). There are community mental health nurses who have a caseload which includes no-one with a diagnosis of schizophrenia (24.5%).

THE DICTATES OF FASHION

By plotting the growth in numbers of nurses and by looking at their work with particular groups, it might be and indeed has been suggested that community mental health nurses are working inappropriately and have shifted the focus of their work away from people with serious and enduring mental illness. We would suggest that the picture is far more complex than this simple explanation allows and that a number of issues must be added to the debate. Firstly, the location of primary health care need not mean refocusing referrals. Secondly, the demands of primary health care need not distract service provision away from people with serious and enduring mental illness. Thirdly, there are individuals who suffer considerably from conditions which do not fall into the category of serious mental illness and schizophrenia and fourthly, the health careers of people who use services have changed with the reprovision of services and the closure of the long-stay mental hospital. As an example, in 1965 for every two admissions to hospital there was one readmission. In 1991 for every one admission to hospital there were two readmissions. There have been 'guesstimates of need' for full provision of service per 100 000 of the population which, it is suggested, might be 40 acute beds, 50 community places and 11 long-term residential places per 100 000. Many community mental health nurses are now located with community mental health teams who will be operating within systems of case management. The reprovision of services and the demands of working in multidisciplinary teams will once again change the work patterns of community mental health nurses.

Unresolved tensions remain between the demands of general practitioners and psychiatrists on the work of nurses.

DEMAND FOR THE SKILLS OF MENTAL HEALTH NURSING IN THE COMMUNITY

There has been a history of specialization and various attempts at advancing the skills of nurses in the last 10–12 year period. The basic skills of mental health nurses have been described in the context of services available to all people with mental illness. A pamphlet published by the Department of Health, *Mental Illness – What Does It Mean?* (1993), has identified the common contribution of the mental health care team as a whole but also the specific core skill which defines and distinguishes the contribution of mental health nursing. It is suggested that doctors, psychologists, nurses, social workers and occupational therapists work as mental health teams in most areas. They have some skills in common, such as counselling, and some that are particular to their individual training and that, in particular, nursing staff are the largest group of trained staff dealing with people with mental health problems. They work in residential settings including psychiatric units and nursing homes and as community psychiatric nurses. Their training equips them with counselling as well as caring, rehabilitation and medication supervision skills. Many nurses have sought to change or improve their skills by specializing in more particular therapies and/or with specific client groups. There is no doubt that nurses are good therapist material but it is important to recognize that core nursing skills have value in their own right which should not be undermined by a constant seeking for alternatives on the assumption that the core skills of mental health nurses are somehow insufficient.

SPECIALIST CLIENT GROUPS

There is some evidence that focusing on particular client groups has allowed the development of positive approaches to care. It is reported that in the United Kingdom 42.1% of community mental health nurses act as specialists. This is a rise of 13% from the preceding five year period. There are now more specialists in rehabilitation and resettlement, which has seen a growth of 12%; however, care of older people is still the largest at 21.3%.

Care of elderly people with mental illness

This is probably the most poorly researched of all the specialist groups; however, nurses specializing with this group are predominantly female and employed at the lower grade points.

It has been suggested (Adams, 1991) that psychoeducational approaches to care with older people may have benefit and screening for depressed people may be a good strategy prior to CPN intervention.

Drug and alcohol misuse

In 1990, 134 specialist community mental health nurses were identified. Anecdotal evidence suggests that this figure is likely to be inaccurate. There is a general lack of training opportunity and career structure for nurses working in the field of substance misuse.

Working with people with HIV and AIDS

Catalan, one of the most prolific authors on the subject (Catalan, 1993), argues that community psychiatric nurses are necessary for people with HIV disease related dementia and this is proving a particular problem for HIV specialist nurses.

Forensic psychiatry

Fifty to sixty specialist services have been reported. One of the most interesting developments in this area in recent times has been the involvement of community mental health nurses in court diversion schemes. Brooker (1991) reports a scheme in which, of the 99 people seen, 50% had a formal psychiatric diagnosis with various interventions. Only three of those 99 reoffended over a two year period.

Liaison work

37% of services in the 1990 survey provided work of this kind. Some interesting work is reported with HIV disease (Jones, 1989) and with other accident and emergency services working with people who have attempted suicide (Atha, 1990).

People with serious and enduring mental illness

Developments with people with serious mental illness, researched by Brooker and Butterworth (1991) at Manchester, have shown that by preparing nurses through a process of careful educational preparation and assessment, changes could be shown in clients which are reflected in a reduction in the severity and frequency of depression, anxiety and retardation. Improvements could be shown in social functioning and a reduction in medication use. The carer showed an improvement in knowledge, consumer satisfaction and social functioning were improved and psychiatric morbidity was reduced.

The promise of case management holds considerable opportunities for community mental health nurses acting as key workers, as does the ten point plan proposed by the Department of Health for successful and safe community care. The care programme approach involves collaboration between health and social services in order that individually tailored care programmes are available for people with mental health problems newly accepted by specialist mental health services and also for people about to be discharged from mental health hospitals. Nurses are increasingly being nominated as key workers which means they are responsible for:

1. collaboration with service users and their carers;
2. acting as a consistent point of contact for service users, carers and other professionals;
3. ensuring that the user is registered with a GP and working in close contact with a primary health care team;
4. ensuring access to health promotion and chronic disease management at a primary health care level;
5. being aware of other resources and referring appropriately;
6. planning and monitoring with others the delivery of the agreed care package, recording decisions made about it and ensuring regular reviews.

The government has also announced a ten-point plan for developing successful and safe community care (DoH, 1993). It has proposed strengthened powers to supervise the care of patients detained under the Mental Health Act who will need special support after they leave hospital. The following have been considered:

1. the period during which patients can be given extended leave and the ability to be recalled to hospital;
2. guidance to ensure that psychiatric patients are not discharged from hospital inappropriately and that those who leave get the right support from different agencies;
3. better training for key workers in their duties under the care programme approach;

4. encouraging the development of better information systems including special supervision registers of patients who may be most at risk;
5. a review of the standards of care for people with schizophrenia both in hospital and in the community and an agreed work programme for the government's Mental Health Task Force ensuring that health authorities and GP fundholder purchasing plans cover the essential needs of mental health services.

It is anticipated that community mental health nurses will take a key role in all these things.

THE WAY FORWARD

Two matters illustrate the debate that will unfold over the next few years and inform the work of the community mental health nurse. Firstly, the focus of work effort. There is now some agreement that the work of mental health nurses must be focused on those people who have an established mental illness; however, other demands are made for mental health care in primary and secondary prevention.

In primary prevention, which has largely to do with reducing the incidence of mental illness, it is suggested by Goldberg and Huxley (1980) that approximately 250 people per 1000 per year are at risk. Community mental health nurses will inevitably give this some attention. It will involve work with vulnerable people or those at most risk of mental illness. This will clearly involve general practitioners, social workers, health visitors, school nurses and practice nurses, health education services and the occasional specialist support of mental health nurses.

In secondary prevention, which is the early detection of mental illness leading to prompt intervention, it is suggested that those at risk are approximately 100 people per 1000 per year. Work is mostly carried out in the primary health care setting, which involves general practitioners, social workers, psychologists, psychiatrists, practice nurses, health visitors and district nurses and requires their continuous liaison with mental health nurses. It will also necessitate some casework by mental health nurses themselves.

Tertiary prevention, which involves treatment and active intervention with established mental illness, suggests that there are 24 people per 1000 per year at risk. It requires early intervention, effective treatment and rehabilitation and a system of active case management, involving psychiatrists, psychologists, social workers, mental health nurses in hospitals, residential facilities, day and community care. It will need occasional support from and work with practice and district nurses.

In this way it is likely that the contribution from community mental health nurses will be refocused in the medium term to manage the demands of more individualized work envisaged by the care programme approach and supervised discharge.

Sustaining and developing community mental health nurses

Community mental health nurses themselves are likely to require a system of support and continuous development which informs and develops their practice. It has been proposed by Butterworth and Faugier (1992) that such a framework is offered by clinical supervision, all the more important given the context of this book. Although the concept of clinical supervision is well accepted in mental health nursing, it is less well established as a reality for most practitioners. It is clear that clinical supervision is certainly not yet the norm for the majority of mental health nurses; for the most part, the only form of clinical supervision to which nurses have access is provided by informal peer group support. There are of course notable exceptions where there has been an attempt to take the issue of clinical supervision seriously, but these examples are few and far between. Clinical supervision can take various forms depending on the philosophy and style of the intervention being offered but it is underpinned by a number of fundamental principles.

1. Skills need to be constantly redefined and improved throughout professional life.
2. Critical discussion about clinical practice is a means to professional development.
3. Introduction to the process of clinical supervision should begin in professional training and continue thereafter as an integral aspect of professional development.

Clinical supervision requires time, energy and commitment. It is not an incidental activity and must be planned and effectively resourced. Clinical supervision has a number of advantages: it places emphasis on the clinical aspects of mental health nursing, it helps nurses to assess their training and research needs, it encourages the recognition and appreciation of individual clients and their social situations and examines multidisciplinary contributions to comprehensive client care. Clinical supervision can identify and develop innovative practice and create an ethos which fosters staff retention and morale and promotes vital links between research and practice. There are, it is argued, three distinct but inter-related aspects of clinical supervision:

1. a formative or educational function which is aimed at developing skills and abilities and understanding of those supervised;
2. a restorative or supportive function which acknowledges the therapeutic use itself and that nurses will be affected by the pain and distress which is suffered by clients. The growth of primary nursing, case management and other person centred approaches will inevitably increase the stresses and the need for clinical supervision which this will involve;
3. a managerial function of supervision supplying external quality control; through this, the supervisor can ensure that the highest professional standards of nursing are upheld.

Clinical supervision is by no means an isolated activity and should be seen in the context of other supportive mechanisms which protect, sustain and develop community mental health nursing, such as continuity in education, performance review and professional development.

REFERENCES

Adams, T. (1991) A family stress model of dementia. *Senior Nurse*, **11**(2), 33–5.

Atha, C. (1990) The role of the CPN with clients who deliberately 1harm themselves, in *Community Psychiatric Nursing – A Research Perspective*, (ed. C. Brooker), Chapman & Hall, London.

Brooker, C. (1991) Position Paper on Community Psychiatric Nursing. University of Manchester.

Brooker, C. and Butterworth, C. (1991) Working with families caring for a relative with schizophrenia: the evolving role of the community psychiatric nurse. *International Journal of Nursing Studies*, **28**(2), 189–200.

Brooker, C. and Simmonds, S. (1985) A study to compare two different models of community psychiatric nursing care delivery. *Journal of Advanced Nursing*, **10**, 217–23.

Butterworth, C. and Faugier, J. (199?) *Clinical Supervision and Mentorship in Nursing*, Chapman & Hall, London.

Carr, P., Butterworth, C. and Hodges, B. (1980) *Community Psychiatric Nursing*, Churchill Livingstone, Edinburgh.

Catalan, J. (1993) HIV Infection and Mental Health Care: Implications for Services. *Second Report of World Health Organisation Regional Office for Europe*.

Department of Health (1993) *Mental Illness – What Does It Mean?* HMSO, London.

Goldberg, D. and Huxley, P. (1980) *Mental Illness in the Community: The Pathway to Psychiatric Care*, Tavistock, London.

Greene, J. (1968) The psychiatric nurse in the community. *International Journal of Nursing Studies*, **5**, 175–83.

Hunter, P. (1974) Community psychiatric nursing in Great Britain: an historical review. *International Journal of Nursing Studies*, **11**, 223–33.

Jones, A. (1989) Liaison consultation psychiatry – the CPN as a clinical nurse specialist. *Community Psychiatric Nursing Journal*, **9**(2), 7–14.

May, A. and Moore, S. (1963) The mental nurse in the community. *Lancet*, **1**, 213–14.

White, E. (1990) *The Third Quinquennial National Community Psychiatric Nursing Survey*, Department of Nursing, University of Manchester.

World Health Organization (1956) Expert Committee in Psychiatric Nursing. Technical Report Series 1–5. WHO, Geneva.

CHAPTER 3

Stress in mental health nursing: a review of the literature

Lynda A. Dunn and Susan A. Ritter

INTRODUCTION

One of the main reasons that stress is so widely researched is the need to understand the role it plays in the onset or maintenance of mechanisms which lead to disease. The assumption is widely accepted that stress, however defined, is a hazard for those employed in the helping or caring professions.

There are two problems associated with the attempt to review the literature on stress and psychiatric and mental health nursing. The first is the lack of explicit links with the psychophysiological literature. The second is the failure of many studies to define operationally the nature of the nursing activities hypothesized to be activators of a stress response. A brief review of major concepts in the stress literature will precede an account of the psychiatric and mental health nursing literature.

Since 1950, the literature on stress can be broadly classified into that which deals with an organism's response to aversive events (stress-as-agent); that which deals with preventing or controlling the effects of such events (stress-as-effect); and that which deals with the nature of the interaction between an individual's psychological, neuroendocrine and behavioural responses (stress-as-transaction). Despite the apparent clarity of such a classification, in practice many workers blur the distinction between stress-as-agent and stress-as-effect (Anisman and Zacharko, 1982; Hamilton and Warburton, 1979).

It is essential that for the purposes of clinical investigation stress-as-agent and stress-as-effect remain clearly distinguished, even though stress-as-transaction may be the assumed and/or preferred model. Clinical observations in the field are subject to almost insurmountable difficulties, which may account for the amount of experimental data on non-human animals. Unless the focus of observation is tightly defined intra- as well as inter-observer reliability is very hard to maintain. There is little agreement among investigators about the reference criteria for measuring severity and intensity of stress-as-agent or stress-as-effect, except in the case of post-traumatic stress disorder. Observations which are not longitudinal and not comparative produce a snapshot effect which may be blurred and which makes the effects of time and individual characteristics hard to interpret.

Even if reference criteria are clearly defined a number of questions remain. Is what is observed a product of the interaction between the observer and the observed? Would a change in circumstances affect things for the worse or for the better? If it seems that all is not well, how can the observer be sure whether this is the worst possible case or a relatively mild case which a change in circumstances could affect very much for the worse or for the better?

STRESS-AS-AGENT

Stress-as-agent is commonly defined in terms of a challenge directed at the organism from its environment. But how is the challenge to be identified and measured? If reference criteria are limited to aversive effects like destruction of one's home, experiencing a road traffic accident or a bereavement, logical problems emerge which are similar to those which have undermined work using life event scales. Events which are widely agreed to be aversive do not produce homogeneous effects in the people who experience them, whether on self-report or by measurement of psychological states. Events which are widely thought of as being agreeable such as promotion at work or retirement from work seem also to be associated with self-reported distress and, in the case of retirement, increased mortality. If reference criteria are limited to direct experience of events, how are threat or the experience of hearing of a traumatic event over the telephone to be classified and measured?

One way round these problems has been to define a challenge as that which activates a physiological response – stress-as-effect.

STRESS-AS-EFFECT

Animal studies have been able to operationalize and classify aversive events according to their timing, nature, duration, intensity and variability. The resulting demands on the animal appear to elicit various responses such as raising nociceptive thresholds, immunosuppression and stomach ulceration, as well as a variety of avoidance behaviours (Watkins and Mayer, 1982). Some responses may be understood as adaptive attempts to cope with the demands of the aversive events. Others are temporary physiopathological alterations in response initially to episodic demands but gradually becoming permanent changes, although the physiological response to a sudden acute episode of stress or shock and its aftermath appears to be different from repetitive or variable demands (Anisman and Zacharko, 1982). Response to acute, chronic, variable, repeated or unrelieved demand appears to be mediated through the neuroendocrine complex, with evidence of links with cardiovascular disease, impaired immunity and, in human beings, episodes of affective and psychotic disorders.

Evidence that depression is mediated by stress must be contrasted with findings which indicate that an episode of depression is better predicted by a previous episode than by the occurrence of an adverse life event. On the other hand, it is possible that physiological changes caused by stressors precipitate a first episode of depression following which depressive responses become self-maintaining (Silvestrini, 1989; Dubovsky, 1990).

What makes stress-as-effect most difficult to measure in human beings is that accurate and specific physiological measures are obtained invasively and by methods that are ethically unacceptable in human respondents; and that accurate and specific measures of mood, such as depression scales, provide material for inferences about the relationship between physiopathology and psychopathology. Causal direction cannot be inferred. For instance, it is commonly assumed that the illness 'depression' is a consequence of altered physiology, so that experiments designed to test this hypothesis risk circularizing any argument in favour of accepting it. Clinical interventions whose rationale is based on a circular argument in turn become impossible to test reliably. If it is hypothesized that the depression alters physiology and thus an individual's appraisal of and response to stress, the consequences for clinicians are somewhat different (Ader and Cohen, 1993).

STRESS-AS-TRANSACTION

Experimental attempts to show that behavioural adaptation or proactive coping moderate physiological responses to stress are complicated by the ways in which individuals appraise potential stressors or threats and the degree to which they avoid or engage with aversive events (Wright, Williams and Dill, 1992). Cognitive psychology has enabled the systematization of a number of common observations. An individual's response to a challenge depends on three factors.

Firstly, he or she will be in a particular physiological state: for example, at its simplest, rested, sleep-deprived, hungry, well-fed, starved. Secondly, he or she will have an appraisal or perception of the threat presented by the challenge: for example, at its simplest, an experienced solo rock climber's appraisal of a cliff face will be different from that of a novice boy scout. Thirdly, he or she will be in a particular psychological state (which is not independent of the first and second factors): either with or without experience of a similar threat or challenge in the past. These three factors may be collapsed into one psychophysiological factor: the individual's state of readiness to undertake tasks or meet a challenge. Readiness will also be constrained when shock or catastrophe bypass conscious appraisal of threat.

A transactional view of stress sees a person representing to themselves an account of the present threat or challenge, the incentives for dealing with it, the likely results of dealing with it, a prediction of what the experience of dealing with it is likely to be (what it will feel like). This view changes the definition of 'environment', because there is some evidence that a person's appraisal of potential threats or challenges may activate neuroendocrine systems. The resulting change in psychophysiological state may alter appraisal of the goals of and incentives for any action, as well as of the threat.

In a review of the psychobiology of post-traumatic stress disorder, van der Kolk and Fisler (1993) describe how the age or developmental stage of an individual affects their response to traumatic stress. The relationship between gender and differences in response to stress in human beings has focused on premenstrual symptoms. An environmental cue for circadian rhythms is known as a **zeitgeber**. Steiner (1992) suggests that the menstrual cycle itself may act as a zeitgeber for women with a history of depression and concurrent psychosocial stress at different stages of their reproductive life. Stages of the menstrual cycle may trigger biological features of the stress response in vulnerable women.

PSYCHIATRIC AND MENTAL HEALTH NURSING

Although stress amongst nurses has been examined in a number of studies, these have mainly focused on general nursing. There is relatively little research into the factors which are important in the field of psychiatric and mental health nursing. A review of the literature reveals that many of the stressors reported by psychiatric nurses are those which are also shared with other types of nursing. Some of the demands facing nurses working in the field of mental health are specific to this field, though they make up few of the overall stressors. For instance, Dawkins *et al.* (1985) used a 78-item Psychiatric Nurses

Occupational Stress Scale which was developed from lists of stressful events reported by nurses. Of the 78 items, only 11 were specific to psychiatric nursing.

The literature also shows that the types of stressor may vary depending on which area of psychiatry a nurse works in. Psychological stress has been examined in nurses working in a special hospital (Graham Jones *et al.*, 1987), in long-stay wards (Landeweerd and Boumans, 1988; Firth *et al.*, 1987), acute admission wards (Sullivan, 1993; Handy, 1990; Landeweerd and Boumans, 1988) and community nursing (Carson *et al.*, 1991; Handy, 1990). Studies within various theoretical frameworks will be discussed briefly.

Psychodynamic perspective

Newnes (1990) suggests that stress is an inevitable feature when large groups of people, such as nurses, need to perform the ill-defined tasks of 'helping people' and 'managing resources'. He proposes that by means of unconscious defence mechanisms, such as projection and denial, staff do not experience extreme anxiety. As a result, assessing actual levels of staff anxiety is extremely difficult. Newnes also suggests that staff sublimate tension through physical sickness and resort to regressive and irresponsible behaviour such as lateness and absenteeism. He reached these conclusions after examining levels of anxiety, depression and hostility experienced by staff in a psychiatric unit and found that scores were no higher than the normal population. Newnes explains his results in terms of a psychodynamic perspective. He argues that staff project their dependency (on higher administration/policies) onto patients and their wish to control and hurt onto the management. Because he does not report any methodological details such as sample size or analysis of data his perspective must be regarded with some caution.

Organizational perspective

During the 1950s and 1960s a number of sociologists in the USA took their fieldwork into mental hospitals. Etzioni's (1960) warning about translating theories such as human relations in industrial settings to the mental hospital has not been widely heeded. Some cross cultural work was carried out in Japan and used to illustrate the nature of the nurse's relationship with mentally ill people. Being a woman and living in special accommodation designed for people who literally spent 24 hours a day with 'their' patients were extremely important factors and are relevant to Nolan's discussion in Chapter 1 (Caudill, 1961). Although they did not describe their work in terms of 'stress', terms like 'morale' were used in order to try to explain features of psychiatric nurses' work, such as hostility towards and withdrawal from patients (Pearlin and Rosenberg, 1962; Meyer, 1967). Baron (1987) describes an anthropological study of a British day hospital which observed high levels of hostility between staff and between staff and patients. The most recent study which used participant observation and focused on occupational stress is by Handy (1990). The reader is referred to Chapter 4 of this book.

Person/environment

Furnham and Walsh (1991) utilized the concept of person/environment fit in their study of 46 psychiatric nurses in Surrey. This theory proposes that there is a need for congruence between a person's personality type and the factors inherent in the work environment. The degree of congruence has been related to stress disorders, job satisfaction and other occupational dependent variables (Holland, 1973). Furnham and Walsh used a self-directed search measure to determine individuals' personality profile and occupation in terms of the framework suggested by Holland (1973). They also used the Job Frustration Questionnaire (Spector, 1975) to assess individuals' level of frustration. Their findings were somewhat surprising in that congruence was negatively correlated with frustration as expected but also positively correlated with absenteeism. There was also no relationship between frustration and absenteeism. The authors gave some possible explanations for this but concluded that the results may have been due to unreliable measures and small sample size, together with the suggestion that nurses may be an idiosyncratic group anyway.

Socialization/transactional perspective

Most of the work within this area is based on an interactionist model of stress in which the role of cognitive events as well as environmental factors is signified in the psychological and physiological response to stressful events. Lazarus and Folkman (1984) describe one of the most well-known interactionist explanations of stress. An individual's appraisal of the causes and consequences of an event is hypothesized to be a significant factor when determining affective and behavioural responses to situations. The appraisal depends on factors such as past experience, familiarity with the situation and past successes or failures.

Davis (1986) examines stress in student psychiatric nurses in terms of the socialization process of nurses: that is, the way in which individuals acquire the knowledge, skills and dispositions that enable them to participate as more or less effective members of groups, organizations or society itself.

BURNOUT

Much of the research on stress in psychiatric nursing also addresses the area of burnout, a term which describes a particular set of psychological responses to stress that is associated with persons working in constant close contact with other people. Although there appears to be little consensus in defining burnout there are certain elements which are shared. Most of the research focuses on the theoretical perspective of Maslach and Jackson (1981) who defined burnout as 'a syndrome of emotional exhaustion, depersonalization and reduced person accomplishment that can occur among individuals who do people work of some kind'. Cherniss (1980) adopted a much wider conceptualization of burnout, referring to 'negative changes in work related attitudes and behaviour in response to job stress'.

Firth *et al.* (1986b) suggest that the concept of 'burnout' has much in common with the concept of professional depression which was a process identified by Oswin (1978) as affecting some nurses in long-stay mental handicap hospitals. Firth *et al.*'s study involved 229 nurses from general and mental handicap hospitals as well as psychiatric units. They used the Maslach Burnout Inventory, the Beck Depression Inventory (BDI) and also a BDI which was adapted to refer to work related items. In the Maslach Inventory the component 'emotional exhaustion' appears to relate closely to the professional depression items which include statements about affect, motivation, perception and behaviour at and about work. The psychometric properties of the scale used to measure professional depression are not reported, so that its reliability and validity cannot be assured. No conclusions can be drawn about the extent to which the results apply to psychiatric nurses, since the distribution of nurses in each setting is not examined.

Burnout and stress have also been related to job satisfaction. Dolan (1987) examined the relationship between burnout and job satisfaction in two groups of recently qualified staff from fields of general and psychiatric nursing. Her sample included 30 psychiatric nurses, 30 general nurses and a control group of 30 administrative staff. Burnout was negatively associated with job satisfaction.

PERSONALITY AND STRESS

A so-called 'stress personality' has been associated with increased neuroticism scores on the Eysenck Personality Inventory (Eysenck and Eysenck, 1964; Krieg *et al.*, 1990). A so-called 'self-defeating personality' has been associated with an external locus of control and with a tendency to regard oneself as a victim (Schill and Beyler, 1992).

Firth *et al.* (1987) used the Bedford and Foulds Personality Deviance Scale (Bedford and Foulds, 1978) to assess the personality of nurses working in long-stay settings and found that personality influenced the type of burnout responses reported. The personality dimension of extrapunitiveness (the tendency to direct hostility and blame onto others) was associated with depersonalization or hardening toward people. On the other hand intropunitiveness (the tendency to project hostility or blame onto oneself) was highly correlated with avoidance of problems and lack of personal accomplishment. Employees who scored higher on either of these dimensions were more likely to report higher levels of discouragement about work.

Jones *et al.* (1987) examined the personality trait of neuroticism as measured using the Eysenck Personality Inventory (Eysenck and Eysenck, 1964). They found that scores on this scale were in fact lower than the normal population and therefore may not have been a major deciding factor in the relatively high levels of reported stress in their sample of nurses.

SOURCES OF STRESS

Most of the events that psychiatric nurses perceived as being stressful identify with the theory of Lazarus and de Longis (1983) in that they describe 'daily hassles': that is, the frequently occurring, irritating and stressful demands of work but not major events/disasters. Lazarus and de Longis suggest that these are more useful in predicting outcomes such as psychological symptoms and somatic illness. The following are sources of stress which psychiatric nurses have identified.

Interpersonal conflict

In the USA Trygstad (1986) found that difficulties in nurse relationships with either other RNs or the head nurse and the ability to work together were the most important determinants of the work stress experienced by psychiatric staff nurses. Her sample consisted of 22 registered psychiatric nurses working on four units of three private hospitals and five units of one federal hospital. It can be seen therefore that each of the units was not well represented. Trygstad conceptualized stress and coping in terms of Lazarus' cognitive appraisal theory and also Selye's (1976) theory of stress and adaptation. Unit staff relationships accounted for one third of all stressors identified. Problems with such relationships included inadequate or ineffective communication and infighting between individuals and groups on the unit. They found that when staff friction did occur both the problem and the distressing feelings often went unresolved.

Problems between unit staff and head nurses accounted for a further 17% of stressors.

Dawkins *et al*. (1985) used a modification of the Holmes and Rahe technique (Holmes and Rahe, 1967) to identify sources of stress in 43 psychiatric nurses. They found that only about a fifth of the job stresses related to staff conflicts. The highest stressors related to working with poorly motivated staff, working with persons who resent new ideas and having others take credit for things which they had worked hard on or initiated. Some of the items that the author placed in the category of 'staff performance' may also be related to interpersonal conflict. For example, 'dealing with the hassle that occurs when you try to take action against incompetent staff' was rated highly as a source of stress. Staff performance accounted for a further 6% of stressors.

In Sullivan's (1993) study interpersonal conflict was found to be rare amongst staff, though when such problems did occur they were described as being very stressful and a major problem.

Organizational factors

Almost invariably in the literature, nurses' perceptions of the organization have been negative. In Sullivan's (1993) study, poor communication, lack of consultation and minimal communication were identified. A central theme in the study was the 'process of change': staff believed there had been no settled period within the last ten years. In Dawkins *et al* 's study all of the top ten stressors identified by nurses referred to administrative/organizational factors. Again change was implicated, including 'not being notified of changes before they occur' and 'working for an administration that believes in change for the sake of change'. Sullivan suggests that such negative conceptions may be due to underlying organizational patterns which may be out of the control of the hospital administration. For example, nurses are functioning in an environment which is characterized by change and insecurity as the shift from hospital to community care takes place. Also sociopolitical policies mean that hospital managers are working within increasing financial constraints. Anomalous results were found in Trygstad's (1986) research whereby only 6% of identified stressors were accounted for by organizational practices. Nurses were particularly frustrated when they perceived that they had no input into the organization.

Patient demands

Jones *et al*. (1987) carried out a study of 349 nurses working in a Special Hospital (response rate of 49%). They looked at the relationships between psychological distress, anxiety and depression as outcomes of the relationship between job demands, supports and constraints. Three major types of job demands were identified: 'administration', 'patient supervision' and 'aversive demands'. Patient supervisory demands were reported to be high though interestingly they were not related to health and well-being. The authors suggested that this was due to nurses' expectancy within their role. Patient supervision is inherent in the role of nurses in a special hospital and so staff expect to spend a large part of their day carrying out this function. Aversive demands which were low were highly associated with psychological distress, anxiety and depression as measured by the General Health Questionnaire (Goldberg and Williams, 1988). In their study nurses were found to have relatively high levels of psychological distress when compared to other employed groups, though not when compared to unemployed samples. In this study 'social attitudes' towards nurses were perceived as a constraint and 'help with patient care' is seen as a support. Communication, administration and union influences could either be a source of support or constraint.

Sullivan (1993) examined occupational stress in 78 nurses in the eight acute admissions wards of two health authorities. Stress was perceived in terms of the theoretical model proposed by Lazarus and Folkman (1984). He also investigated the stress outcome of burnout, using the Maslach Burnout Inventory. He developed a Psychiatric Nurse Stress Inventory which scored stress on five subscales: patient care; work environment; interpersonal conflict; support, and perceptions of the organization. The most frequent stressors relating to patient care were violent incidents, potential suicide and observation. He found that the perceived predictability and availability of adequate nursing staff influenced the intensity of the stress. High scores on patient care stressors were associated with emotional exhaustion. Staffing problems were found to relate to both the numbers of staff and competence, motivation and suitability of relief staff. High scores relating to staffing, administrative duties and work overload were also found to correlate with increased levels of emotional exhaustion. In the study approximately 45% of nurses scored high on emotional exhaustion and depersonalization and only about 14% showed high scores on the personal accomplishment subscale which measures positive levels of personal accomplishment.

Trygstad (1986) found that problems with patients accounted for 13% of stressors. Patient chronicity and recidivism in particular were described frequently by nurses as sources of stress. Negative patient characteristics accounted for only 9% of stressors in Dawkins *et al.*'s (1985) research, with 'a physical threat by a patient' being the only one scoring high on stressfulness.

Violence by patients

Whittington (1992) conducted a series of studies in a mental illness hospital, first examining the extent and effects of violence by patients towards nurses, then the effect of moderating variables. He found that apparently minor episodes of violence could precipitate periods of absence from work, as well as prolonged feelings of dysphoria. Social support was a strong moderator of adverse effects of violence.

Rix (1987) examined the relationship between staff sickness and violence in a regional secure unit, finding that, while violence by patients was associated with feelings of vulnerability and frustration in nurses who also went off sick, levels of absenteeism were moderated by complex organizational and dispositional factors among the nurses.

The findings of Cairns and Wilson (1989) concerning violence in Northern Ireland may be relevant to nurses' experience of violence by patients. They suggest that denial is a main coping strategy and that this in turn is related to an individual's appraisal of violence rather than to their disposition or personality.

HOW STRESS IS MODERATED

In addition to the potential stressors within psychiatric nursing the role of 'moderating' variables has been studied.

A relationship between social support and stress has been observed for a long time and it has been suggested by Michaels (1971) that nurses are often so in need of support themselves that they are unable to give support to their patients. This would seem of particular import-ance to nurses working in psychiatry whose primary role often necessitates giving support to patients. Firth *et al.* (1986a) suggest that staff support can be viewed both in terms of organizational support and interpersonal support. The former comprises factors such as resources, staff, training and management structure and the latter refers to support that staff get through face-to-face contact with other people. Studies within this area have tended to concentrate on the second of the two: interpersonal support.

Cronin-Stubbs and Brophy (1984) examined the relationship between social support, occupational stress and life stress. They compared nurses working in various work settings, 66 of whom worked in psychiatry. Social support was found to be negatively associated with and predictive of burnout. Working within the field of psychiatry was also found to be predictive of burnout. This was a reflection of the intense interpersonal involvement and conflict (which were positively associated with burnout) that the nurses described experiencing.

Psychiatric nurses also experienced less affirmation than other nurses, both on and off the job. Cronin-Stubbs and Brophy (1984) attributed this to the fact that psychiatric nurses' interventions are less observable than those of general nurses because most care occurs as nurse–patient interactions. They also suggested that psychiatric nurses may avoid intense personal contact at home. Affect and emotional support were both found to be negatively and significantly associated with burnout.

Firth *et al.* (1986a) also examined the relationship of social support to burnout as well as eliciting from nurses their perceptions of supportive behaviour in their superiors. Cherniss (1980) describes three components of support: feedback on performance; information, advice or technical assistance; and emotional support or ventilation of feelings. Firth *et al.* (1986a) identified five factors which indicated a helpful relationship. These were:

1. Personal respect. This was concerned with availability and approachability as well as feedback, information-giving, encouragement and thanks.
2. Empathic attention. This comprised attending to, understanding and reflecting others' concerns.
3. Absence of interpersonal defensiveness and lack of straightforward interpersonal communication.
4. Absence of indignation or impatience.
5. Concern for feelings. This was related to empathy concerning staff feelings.

The attributes which made up personal respect and empathetic attention were found to be observable and rateable by staff as shown by inter-rater reliability scores. However, the other factors did not seem to be as tangible, a factor which Firth *et al.* (1986a) interpreted as reflecting staff's own perceptions or specific aspects of interpersonal interactions. Perceived level of support was also found to be significantly related to reduced emotional exhaustion, depersonalization and fewer thoughts of leaving.

There was some evidence that aspects of support are 'passed through the hierarchy'. Staff who reported feelings of depersonalization in their work were reported as showing less personal respect to their subordinates. Firth *et al.* (1986b) also found that role clarity and the degree of personal face-to-face contact with a superior were important influences on 'professional depression', emotional draining and depersonalization.

Whittington and Wykes (1992) examined social support in 24 psychiatric nurses with regard to a specific incident, that of assault by a patient. Violence or the threat of violence from patients is a problem widespread in psychiatric nursing and one which has been cited as a significant source of stress. The assaults studied were mostly 'minor' in that there was no physical injury, but this is the type of violence that nurses are most frequently subjected to. The authors found that despite the impact of an assault lasting for several weeks in some cases, support in terms of opportunities to talk about the event was only available for a very short period of time after the incident. Most of the support offered was also on an informal basis, for example at home or with colleagues, and over half the victims said they were not completely satisfied with the support they received.

Sullivan's (1993) findings suggest that nurses in his study perceived organizational support as ineffective and that ward teams formed quite an important source of support. This finding is similar to those of the nurses in Trygstad's (1986) study which indicated that co-workers provided 42% of nurses' support. The head nurse provided a further 27% of all support to the staff.

EFFECTS OF NURSES' STRESS ON PATIENTS

Only one study has specifically looked at the effects of staff stress on patients. Gray and Diers (1992) carried out a retrospective study of the effects of the merger of two neuropsychiatric units. They examined how patients' behaviour may be affected by the characteristics of the system and by nurses' behaviour and feelings such as low morale. The findings were paradoxical in that during periods when staff were least stressed and reported being in control of their stress, acute patient behaviours such as requirement for and duration of individual nursing care, use of the quiet room, seclusion and restraints appeared to peak. The authors concluded that this was possibly due to increased attentiveness or more control by staff of unit functioning. Another possible reason cited was that patients may have sensed that their 'acting out' behaviour could be dealt with by staff and safety maintained. This study was unfortunately flawed by incomplete, retrospective data.

Cronin-Stubbs and Brophy (1984) found a relationship between stress and nurses' behaviour with regard to patient care. They found that nurses with higher burnout scores tended to use prescription drugs to calm down patients and spent less time in direct contact with them. These findings could be explained in terms of the need for control during times of personal stress and the inability to maintain support to patients.

COMMUNITY PSYCHIATRIC NURSING

Despite the move from institutional to community care there has not been a wide focus on stress in community psychiatric nursing.

Much of the existing work is summarized elsewhere in this book and will not be repeated here.

DRAWBACKS OF THE RESEARCH

The research within this particular area is limited by various methodological problems. Most of the samples in the research are very small and apply only to specific areas of psychiatry. In fact, many of the studies only examine psychiatric nursing as a subset within their research. This limits the generalizability of the findings (though it is interesting that common sources of stress are often found).

The measures used are often based on self-report and it has been suggested that nurses are socialized not to admit to feelings of strain (Marshall, 1980). In any case, self-report data are based upon the nurses' own perceptions and other influencing variables are not identified.

Another problem in all of the studies is a lack of knowledge about those who did not take part. It is therefore not known whether there are differences in the feelings of those who chose not to take part in the research. There was, as is often the case in research on nurses, a low response rate. For example, Moores and Grant (1977) found that questionnaire response rates were associated with nurses' felt participation in decision making. It may be that respondents were those that felt particularly stressed and wished to make their feelings known. Conversely, stress may have led to disaffection and so to a poor response rate.

Where data were collected by means of interview, the subjectivity of the researchers needs to be taken into account. In a study where nurses were required to keep a record of their activities/feelings, results were limited by inconsistent record keeping and lost data (Gray and Diers, 1992).

Much of the research, as previously mentioned, examines stress in relation to the outcome of burnout using the Maslach Burnout Inventory. Dolan (1987) has criticised the MBI for its 'subtle, ambiguous and vague statements'. She says that measurements of burnout should include factors such as decreasing self-esteem, self-hopelessness, cynicism, negativism and self-depletion.

It was suggested at the start of this chapter that even though stress-as-transaction may be the assumed and/or preferred model investigators must distinguish between stress-as-agent and stress-as-effect and that unless the focus of observations in the field is tightly defined, observer reliability is hard to maintain. Unless the same measures of severity and intensity of stress are consistently used, comparison between studies is difficult. In the case of post-traumatic stress disorder following single incidents, investigators in the UK are encouraged to use as their core measures the GHQ-28, the Impact of Event Scale (Horowitz *et al.*, 1979) and the revised 90-item Symptom Checklist (Derogatis, 1977). This means that investigators can be increasingly confident that they are measuring what they think they are measuring and that data concerning individuals' responses to traumatic stress, as well as their responses to treatment, can be accumulated. The methods and results of the studies of psychiatric and mental health nursing reviewed here are not consistent enough to make firm inferences about working practices. Nor are there any follow-up data.

Perhaps the most worrying deficit is the absence of empirical data about the effect that such stress as reported in the literature has on patient care. The sociological studies of the 1950s and the 1960s and Handy's more recent work (Chapter 4) suggested a link between hostility towards patients and low morale among nurses in psychiatric hospitals. Reports of ill treatment of patients in British hospitals have been tentatively linked to post-traumatic stress disorder in nurses who served during the Second World War (Chapter 1). Relationships between psychiatric and mental health nurses' stress (however defined) and outcomes of nursing care urgently need to be studied.

REFERENCES

Ader, R. and Cohen, N. (1993) Psychoneuroimmunology: conditioning and stress. *Annual Review of Psychology*, **44**, 53–85.

Anisman, H. and Zacharko, R. (1982) Depression: the predisposing influence of stress. *Behavioural and Brain Sciences*, **5**, 89–137.

Baron, C. (1987) *From Asylum to Anarchy*, Free Association Books, London.

Bedford, A. and Foulds, G. (1978) *Personality Deviance Scale (Manual)*, NFER Publishing Co, Windsor.

Cairns, E. and Wilson, R. (1989) Coping with political violence in Northern Ireland. *Social Science and Medicine*, **28**, 621–4.

Carson, J., Bartlett, H. and Croucher, P. (1991) Stress in community psychiatric nursing: a preliminary investigation. *Community Psychiatric Nursing Journal*, **11**, 8–12.

Caudill, W. (1961) Around the clock patient care in Japanese psychiatric hospitals: the role of the Tsukisoi. *American Sociological Review*, **26**, 204–14.

Cherniss, C. (1980) *Professional Burnout in Human Service Organisations*, Praeger, New York.

Cronin-Stubbs, D. and Brophy, E.B. (1984) Burnout: can social support save the psychitric nurse? *Journal of Psychosocial Nursing in Mental Health Services*, **23**, 8–13.

Davis, B. (1986) The strain of training: being a student psychiatric nurse, in *Psychiatric Nursing Research*, (ed. J. Brooking), John Wiley and Sons, Chichester.

Dawkins, J.E., Depp, F. and Selzer, N. (1985) Stress and the psychiatric nurse. *Journal of Psychosocial Nursing*, **23**(11), 9–15.

Derogatis, L. R. (1977) *SCL-90R: Administration Scoring and Procedures Manual*. Clinical Psychometric Research, Baltimore.

Dolan, N. (1987) The relationship between burnout and job satisfaction in nurses. *Journal of Advanced Nursing*, **12**, 3–12.

Dubovsky, S.L. (1990) Understanding and treating depression in anxious patients. *Journal of Clinical Psychiatry*, **51** (Supplement) 3–8, 14–17.

Etzioni, A. (1960) Interpersonal and social factors in the study of mental hospitals. *Psychiatry*, **23**, 13–22.

Eysenck, H.J. and Eysenck, S.B.G. (1964) *Manual of the Eysenck Personality Inventory*, London University Press, London.

Firth, H., McIntee, J., McKeown, P. and Britton P. (1986a) Interpersonal support amongst nurses at work. *Journal of Advanced Nursing*, **11**, 273–82.

Firth, H., McIntee, J., McKeown, P. and Britton P. (1986b) Burnout and professional depression: related concepts? *Journal of Advanced Nursing*, **11**, 633–41.

Firth, H., McIntee, J., McKeown, P. and Britton P. (1987) Burnout, personality and support in long-stay nursing. *Nursing Times*, **83** (32), 55–7.

Furnham, A. and Walsh, J. (1991) Consequences of person–environment incongruence: absenteeism, frustration and stress. *Journal of Social Psychology*, **131** (2), 187–204.

Goldberg, D. and Williams, P. (1988) *A User's Guide to the General Health Questionnaire*, NFER-Nelson, Windsor.

Gray, S. and Diers, D. (1992) The effect of staff on patient behaviour. *Archives of Psychiatric Nursing*, **6** (1), 26–34.

Hamilton, V. and Warburton, D. (eds) (1979) *Human Stress and Cognition*, John Wiley and Sons, Chichester.

Handy, J. (1990) *Occupational Stress in a Caring Profession: The Social Context of Psychiatric Nursing*, Avebury, Aldershot.

Holland, J. (1973) *Making Vocational Choices: A Theory of Careers*. Prentice-Hall, New York.

Holmes, T.H. and Rahe, R.H. (1967) The social readjustment rating scale. *Journal of Psychosomatic Research*, **11**, 213–18.

Horowitz, M., Wilner, N. and Alvarez, W. (1979) The Impact of Events Scale. *Psychosomatic Medicine*, **41**, 209–18.

Jones, J., Janman, K., Payne, R. and Rick, J. (1987) Some determinants of stress in psychiatric nurses. *International Journal of Nursing Studies*, **24**, 129–44.

Krieg, J.C., Lauer, C.J., Hermle, L. *et al.* (1990) Psychometric, polysomnographic, and neuroendocrine measures in subjects at high risk for psychiatric disorders. *Neuropsychobiology*, **23** (2), 57–67.

Landeweerd, J.A. and Boumans, N.P.G. (1988) Nurses' work satisfaction and feelings of health and stress in three psychiatric departments. *International Journal of Nursing Studies*, **25** (3), 225–34.

Lazarus, R.S. and de Longis, A. (1983) Psychological stress and coping in aging. *American Psychologist*, **38**, 245–54.

Lazarus, R.S. and Folkman, S. (1984) *Stress, Appraisal and Coping*, Springer, New York.

Marshall, J. (1980) Stress amongst nurses, *White Collar and Professional Stress*, (eds C.L. Cooper and J. Marshall), John Wiley and Sons, New York.

Maslach, C. and Jackson, S. (1981) The measurement of experienced burnout. *Journal of Occupational Behaviour*, **2**, 99–113.

Meyer, J. (1967) Collective disturbances and staff organization on psychiatric wards. *Sociometry* **30**, 180 99.

Michaels, D.R. (1971) Too much in need of support to give any? *American Journal of Nursing*, **71**, 1932–5.

Moores, B. and Grant, G.W.B. (1977) Feelings of alienation among nursing staff in hospitals for the mentally handicapped. *International Journal of Nursing Studies*, **14**, 5–12.

Newnes, C. (1990) Caring for carers' needs. *Nursing*, **4** (16), 33–4.

Oswin, M. (1978) *Children Living In Long Stay Hospitals*, Heinemann, London.

Pearlin, L.I. and Rosenberg, M. (1962) Nurse–patient social distance and the structural context of a mental hospital. *American Sociological Review*, **27**, 56–65.

Rix, G. (1987) Staff sickness and its relationship to violent incidents in a regional secure unit. *Journal of Advanced Nursing*, **12**, 223–8.

Schill, T. and Beyler, J. (1992) Self-defeating personality and strategies for coping with stress. *Psychological Reports*, **71**(1), 67–70.

Selye, H. (1976) *The Stress of Life*, McGraw Hill, New York.

Silvestrini, B. (1989) Trazodone: from the mental pain to the 'dys-stress' hypothesis of depression. *Clinical Neuropharmacology*, **12** (Supplement 1), S4–10.

Spector, P. (1975) Relationships of organizational frustration with reported behavioural reactions of employees. *Journal of Applied Psychology*, **60**, 635–7.

Steiner, M. (1992) Female-specific mood disorders. *Clinical Obstetrics and Gynaecology*, **35**(3), 599–611.

Sullivan, P.J. (1993) Occupational stress in psychiatric nursing. *Journal of Advanced Nursing*, **18**, 591–601.

Trygstad, L.N. (1986) Stress and coping in psychiatric nursing. *Journal of Psychosocial Nursing*, **24**(10), 23–7.

Van der Kolk, B.A. and Fisler, R.E. (1993) The biologic basis of post-traumatic stress. *Primary Care*, **20**(2), 417–32.

Watkins, L. and Mayer, D. (1982) Organisation of endogenous opiate and nonopiate pain control systems. *Science*, **216** (4551), 1185–92.

Whittington, R. (1992) PhD thesis London University. Institute of Psychiatry.

Whittington, R. and Wykes, T. (1992) Staff strain and social support in a psychiatric hospital following assault by a patient. *Journal of Advanced Nursing*, **17**, 480–6.

Wright, R. Williams, B. and Dill, J. (1992) Interactive effects of difficulty and instrumentality of avoidant behaviour on cardiovascular reactivity. *Psychophysiology*, **29**(6), 677–86.

CHAPTER 4

Stress in mental health nursing: a sociopolitical analysis

Jocelyn Handy

INTRODUCTION

This chapter examines the relationship between the structure and ideology of the mental health system and the occupational stresses experienced by mental health nurses. In so doing, it complements and extends the insights provided by several earlier studies of psychiatry which have sought to illustrate the problems which the psychiatric system creates for those who enter it as patients (Goffman, 1971; Baruch and Treacher, 1978; Baron, 1987) Valuable and disturbing as these critiques are, they only address one half of the problem, for they generally fail to acknowledge that staff, as well as patients, may experience distress as a result of their involvement with the mental health establishment. The dynamics of the psychiatric system are not those of 'oppressors and oppressed' but of an institution manifestly failing to meet the human needs of both those it exists to help and those who labour within it. As this chapter will try and show, the problems of staff are inextricably linked to the experiences of patients and, in consequence, the occupational stresses which they face cannot be fully understood without interpreting the various ways in which the mental health system structures the lives of all who participate within it.

In recent years, the occupational problems besetting the various caring professions have become a prominent concern within the burgeoning literatures on occupational stress and burnout (Pines and Maslach, 1978; Cherniss, 1980; Payne and Firth, 1987; Wallis and de Wolff, 1988). Unfortunately, these literatures tend to concentrate on the perspective of staff without interpreting either the inter-relationship between the experiences of care givers and recipients or the ways in which the social context of care influences all participants' interpretations of their situation. As a result, these literatures tend to underestimate the complexity of people's relationship to their environment and oversimplify the problems which they face (Handy, 1988; Newton, 1989). In order to gain a deeper understanding of the problems of occupational stress within the mental health system we must move beyond the microlevel analyses advocated in traditional stress research and develop more complex interpretations which tackle the interaction between the mental health system's social role and the subjective experiences of those who work within it.

The rest of this chapter is divided into four sections. The first section examines recent sociological writing within the field of critical psychiatry. Theorists within this area have paid relatively little attention to the occupational problems of mental health professionals and have tended to be highly critical of staff whenever they have considered their actions. However, these critics have analysed the functions and structures of the mental health system in some depth and their writings can therefore be drawn upon to develop a richer understanding of the complex relationship between the structural and ideological dimensions of the mental health system and the work experiences of mental health nurses. The second section describes the research setting and methodology. The two succeeding sections present the empirical data and document the ways in which the collective coping strategies employed by mental health nurses in both the hospital and community settings could have the unintended consequence of recreating many of the more pernicious aspects of organizational life within the mental health system and exacerbating the very problems that the nurses were attempting to solve.

CRITICAL PSYCHIATRY

All societies have a tendency to respond to the disturbed or disturbing behaviours of individuals by developing various socially legitimated practices aimed at making such acts more comprehensible to and controllable by their members. The form which such practices take varies widely, for different societies interpret and deal with the same behaviours in divergent ways. Within Western society, the mental health system is an important mechanism for dealing with some forms of socially problematic or personally distressing behaviour.

The most recent literature within the field of critical psychiatry has tended to argue that the mental health system serves a dual purpose within modern society and exists both to help the troubled individual and to supply corrective measures where an individual's behaviour is seen as socially disruptive in some way. This means that the mental health system plays an important role in helping to formulate and to maintain social values and it may in a real sense help to determine socially accepted parameters of mental health or illness (Busfield, 1986; Conrad and Schneider, 1980; Horowitz, 1982; Ingleby, 1981, 1985; Mangen, 1982; Miller and Rose, 1986; Morgan, 1975; Penfold and Walker, 1984; Scheper-Hughes and Lovell, 1986; Turner, 1987).

Theorists who analyse the mental health system from this perspective usually highlight three key problems facing the mental health establishment. The first and most important problem is that the mental health system is simultaneously part of the ideological and regulatory superstructure of industrialized society and an institution which aims to alleviate the personal distress which that society and its institutions help produce. A second and lesser problem is that the mental health system is simultaneously committed to the alleviation of mental illness and to identifying increasingly subtle behavioural deviations and personal distress as mental health problems. The third problem is that the concept of mental illness simultaneously removes individual responsibility for their actions from the patients and makes compliance with professional advice a prerequisite of appropriate patient behaviour. Each of these issues will now be looked at in greater detail.

The most important problem identified in virtually all the recent critiques of the mental health system centres on the tension between, and the interweaving of, the system's dual mandate for helping the individual and ensuring social regulation. The basic argument is that the mental health system has a tendency to locate the sources of people's problems within either organic dysfunctions or psychological dysfunctions within the individual or their immediate family and by so doing it implicitly denies the relationship between social conditions and human experience. This often leads to treatment goals which aim to adjust the individual to a lifestyle compatible with psychiatric definitions of normality. Since these definitions are derived from prevailing cultural norms, psychiatry helps to legitimate the existing social structure both by diverting attention away from competing explanations which emphasize the relationship between individual distress and social conditions and by adjusting individuals to the circumstances in which they live. The effects of this may be detrimental for patients as alternative perspectives and solutions are obscured. For many critics the mental health system is thus a Janus-faced institution whose tremendous potential for helping the individual is too often misdirected towards obscuring the social origins of much physical and mental suffering.

The second problem identified within the critical psychiatry literature centres on the idea that the mental health system is simultaneously committed to the alleviation of mental illness and to identifying increasingly subtle forms of behavioural deviation and personal distress as problems needing the expert intervention of mental health professionals. Several theorists argue that the remit of mental health care has altered radically since the early days of psychiatry (Castel *et al.*, 1982; Eaton, 1986; Ramon, 1985; Scheper-Hughes and Lovell, 1987). Whilst the early psychiatrists were primarily concerned with the incarceration of highly disturbed individuals, the modern mental health establishment often deals with mildly difficult or distressed individuals who are still living within the community. In consequence, the former rigid barriers between mental illness and normality have become permeable. The effect of this, however, is less to remove the stigma of mental illness from severely disturbed individuals and more to suggest that nearly every aspect of life has pathological elements which would benefit from expert adjustment. In other words, modern psychiatry involves the pathologization of normality rather than the eradication of mental illness. This can be seen in the accelerating expansion of psychiatric categories and in the extension of the mental health system to new areas such as childhood behaviour problems, sexual dysfunction and addictions.

The final problem identified within the critical psychiatry literature centres on the equivocal implications of mental health intervention for individual responsibility. As many writers have pointed out, the cultural definition of mental illness has logically inconsistent implications for the issue of personal responsibility (Bott, 1976; Scott, 1973). On the one hand, cultural norms concerning mental illness highlight the concepts of unintelligibility and lack of responsibility, whilst on the other hand norms concerning appropriate sick role behaviour give patients a clear duty to comply with medical treatment. As a result, various paradoxes and ambiguities are created in the relationship between patients, their families and mental health professionals. All parties within the mental health system tend to collude in denying these issues and by doing so they help maintain a system where key therapeutic concerns remain unexamined. This enables patients and their families to exploit the contradictions of the mental health system in order to avoid taking responsibility for their actions, maintain the status quo and obtain relief from the consequences of their actions, whilst simultaneously giving staff a mandate to deny the validity of the patient's perspective whenever it conflicts with their own goals. Unfortunately, the short-term gains which all parties obtain from this strategy are frequently offset by longer term costs which may be devastating.

Recent writing in the critical psychiatry literature suggest that the mental health sector fulfils a complex and ambivalent social function, serving as a key ideological and regulatory mechanism of modern society and as a primary resource for alleviating the misery in our society. This perspective is seldom part of the world view of the various mental health professions, who are socialized into conceptualizing themselves as providers of a therapeutic service based upon growing professional expertise and objectively validated knowledge. For them, the problems of the mental health system are those of inadequate funding, competing philosophies of treatment and poor training. Real as these problems are, in the view of many of psychiatry's critics they are only a part of the problem, for in the final analysis it is the social role of the mental health system which undermines the often very genuine attempts of mental health professionals to help their patients. From this perspective, the negative effects of the mental health system on staff and patients will not be wholly understood unless we locate the subjective experiences of all participants within a wider analysis of the system's relationship to modern society. Only by doing so can we gain real insights into the stresses which the various mental health professionals face.

The succeeding sections of this chapter will now move from the level of abstract theorizing to a grounded analysis of daily life within the mental health system. As the empirical research which follows will reveal, the attempts of different participants to ameliorate the chronic personal insecurities engendered by the structural contradictions of the mental health system often have the paradoxical effect of augmenting their problems and intensifying the very feelings they are struggling to avoid.

METHODOLOGY

The empirical research described in this chapter sought to link the patterns of daily life within the mental health system to the theoretical analysis of the system's ambivalent role within modern society. This necessitated using a research design and methodology which could illuminate the ways in which social structure can influence both people's daily activities and their interpretations of their social circumstances. Such processes are complex and can only be studied by developing a research strategy with enough flexibility to provide a holistic and detailed view of the unfolding of the mental health process over time. In order to accomplish this the research was therefore designed as an indepth case study which used a variety of techniques capable of tapping different aspects of social life.

The research was designed as a comparative study of nursing stress within both the hospital setting and the community. The actual units studied were an acute admissions ward and a community mental health nursing service attached to the same hospital. The various research techniques were chosen firstly because they enabled different facets of the research problem to be investigated in a theoretically meaningful way and secondly because they provided corroborative evidence of the validity and reliability of data. Table 4.1 gives a description of the strengths and limitations of the various techniques used.

Table 4.1 Summary of aims and techniques

Aim	Technique	Strengths	Limitations
To collect data concerning nurses' tacit knowledge and daily activities within the organizational setting	Participant observation Diaries Ward Kardex comments	Direct record of activity within organization	Participant observation is ill-defined data set. All techniques yield highly complex data requiring interpretation by researcher
To collect data concerning nurses' discursive knowledge/feelings about work	Diaries Depth interviews	Direct record of nurses' reflexive knowledge concerning work	Interview reports of action not equivalent to direct observation
To collect numerical data on quantifiable aspects of unit structure	Official statistics Activity schedules Kardex	Clearly defined data sets allow frequency and distribution of events to be calculated	Does not yield information linking patterns with symbols or meanings underlying behaviour

This research strategy enabled the strengths and weaknesses of the different techniques to be counterbalanced and a more complete picture of organizational life developed.

As the empirical data reported in the next two sections will reveal, one of the clearest findings which emerged from the use of this research strategy was that the various contradictions of the mental health sector were repeatedly reflected in discrepancies between the various participants' actual behaviour and their verbal justifications for these acts.

THE ADMISSIONS WARD

General description

This ward was a mixed sex short-stay admissions unit for 30 patients who were admitted to the ward by five consultant psychiatrists. The main criterion for admission to the ward was the geographical location of the patient's home rather than the type of problems presented and, as a result, the ward usually contained a wide range of patients with very disparate problems. The official statistics showed that the average length of stay on the ward was six weeks, although the length varied from a few days to several months. Approximately two thirds of the patients were readmissions and the ward seemed to serve a relatively small population who reappeared rather regularly over the years.

The ward was run by eight permanent day staff plus a fluctuating but roughly equivalent number of trainees. There were generally four nurses on duty per shift, although very often only the most senior staff member was fully qualified. The daily pattern of nursing activities on the ward centred on control and was geared to the routine care of patients' physical needs within a medically oriented treatment regime which placed patients in a passive and dependent role in relation to the staff.

The core treatment programme on the ward was chemotherapy and all patients were given regular medication, which came to symbolize treatment for many of them. Since medication was prescribed by doctors and merely dispensed by nurses the ward became, for many patients, a place where they waited for treatment to occur rather than an integral part of their treatment programme. The nurses tended to administer drugs routinely, without giving much thought to either the symbolic meaning of treating patients with drugs or the physical effects of drugs on the nervous system and there were many occasions where staff linked the passivity and social ineptness of patients to their mental illnesses or personalities without considering the influence of either the ward environment or their medication on the patients' actions.

Despite this, the nurses did have a sense of commitment to the patients' general welfare and the younger nurses would often choose to go and sit with patients and try and converse with them. These interactions were generally initiated on an ad hoc basis when a nurse had some free time and were often difficult for both patients and nurses, partly because the hospital environment was relatively depriving for patients and they therefore had little to talk and partly because the general atmosphere of the smoke filled ward lounge with its constantly blaring television inevitably limited conversation to superficial topics. Not surprisingly, the nurses tended to terminate these conversations after relatively brief periods and to retire to the security of the nursing office and the company of other staff.

The nurses' diaries

The problems which a control oriented ward structure geared to an organic model of mental illness could create for both staff and patients can be illustrated by examining a brief extract from the diary of a student nurse (Figure 4.1). This document reveals some of the ways

Nurse's description of events	Nurse's comments
Admitted another lady, an old patient I've known from the past. Hypomaniac - also suffers from mood swings. Believes in San Yasin (orange people). Neglected hygiene, stopped eating. Varying emotions - crying - laughing - screaming.	Mad at the thought of admitting this lady again as it has only been six weeks since her discharge. Always admitted when her bisexual boyfriend has found another girlfriend. X cannot cope with this - always plays the psychiatric role and always warrants admission. Since her arrival has been kissing walls, lifting clothes up in the lounge. Counselled her re this but to little effect. Maintains it is through (boyfriend) she has ended up coming in. Given prescribed injection to calm her.

Figure 4.1 Diary excerpt of a student nurse.

in which the contradictions of the psychiatric system manifest themselves in the nurses' relationships with patients in a manner which the nurses subjectively experienced as quite stress provoking.

The patient described in this excerpt was an ex-school teacher in her early 30s who had been diagnosed as manic depressive and was being treated within an organic model involving the long-term administration of lithium salts. The patient definitely exhibited quite severe mood swings and was generally admitted to hospital in either a manic state in which she displayed the sort of disinhibited behaviour described by the nurse or a very withdrawn state in which she neglected her hygiene and eating and remained mute. Whilst these symptoms may have had an organic basis, the nurse's comments indicate that the patient's behaviour also seemed to be influenced by a number of social factors which were not being dealt with because her problem was officially conceptualized in biological terms. In this instance, the main precipitant of a severe mood swing seemed to be a serious row with her boyfriend which had involved him threatening to leave her. The patient's hospitalization had always reconciled the couple and provided them with a needed respite in which to renegotiate their relationship. However, it also escalated the inherent problems within the relationship by enabling him to justify his behaviour by locating their problems within her madness and enabling her to precipitate an admission whenever she felt the relationship was in danger. The long-term effect of this was that the hospital had become involved in their relationship as a third party which simultaneously bound the couple together and made their relationship more unstable by ensuring that both partners could relinquish responsibility for their acts and blame the patient's illness for the problems in their relationship.

Although the patient could, perhaps, have behaved more rationally than a purely organic interpretation of her illness would imply, her behaviour was probably not a deliberate dissimulation. What appeared to happen was that the social context which she inhabited facilitated certain forms of behaviour which were irrational by normal standards and which remained incomprehensible to both the patient and staff because they failed to analyse her actions within the social context of the mental health system.

The nurse's description of this patient indicates that she experienced some confusion and frustration about this case. While she was obviously aware of the effect of the patient's personal relationship on her behaviour, she did not seem to consider the effects of the more general mental health context beyond claiming that the patient always 'plays the sick role' to manipulate an admission. This statement then seemed to strike the nurse as too extreme and she immediately qualified it by affirming in another part of her diary that the patient had 'genuine mood swings' which were stabilized through lithium. The nurse's attempts to explain the patient's behaviour thus oscillated rapidly between an individually oriented psychological model in which the patient took full responsibility for her actions and a medical model in which the patient had no responsibility. The nurse's attempts to control the patient's behaviour revealed similar inconsistencies. She initially tried to quieten the patient through verbal remonstrance but then resorted to a medical model and asked the doctor to prescribe a tranquillizing injection. She later commented to me, rather bitterly, that the patient 'was never satisfied until she's proved she's ill by making you give her an injection'.

The remarks of the nurse thus seem to indicate that she felt trapped into acts she felt uncomfortable with for reasons she was unsure of. The nurse's descriptions of her interactions with other patients illustrated the same problems and indicated that the paradoxes of the mental health system coloured most of her relationships with them.

The interview data

The interview data provided further insights into the ways in which the paradoxes of the mental health system could trap the nurses into actions which they felt quite ambivalent about and which they subjectively experienced as quite distressing. During their interviews many of the nurses expressed an uneasy awareness of the discrepancies between the official ideology of the mental health system and their daily activities on the ward. The younger nurses, in particular, often expressed concern about the control oriented ethos of their daily activities and spoke of their desire to develop more effective therapeutic relationships with patients. They often tried to do this by singling out a few specific patients for special attention. Unfortunately, the wider environment of the mental health system often doomed these attempts to failure. When this happened the nurses often reacted quite defensively and blamed patients for lacking the motivation to change, without examining the wider context in which the patients' acts took place. For example, one of the staff nurses described a patient she had once tried to help with the words:

> These days I find I really dislike X. I was quite enthusiastic with her when she first came in – but she's sort of squashed me flat with negative answers every time I came up with something that I felt might be quite good for her ... she knows her problems and she knows the answers – she's just not doing anything about it – she prefers to be the sick person, the person with the problems – so these days I try and avoid her because I find it quite frustrating.

These actions and attributions were often subtly encouraged by the more experienced staff, who tended to reinforce the younger nurses's incipient cynicism even while they paid lip service to the ideal of more individualized care. Ironically, one of the key stratagems for controlling nurses who seemed to be deviating from socially acceptable norms was to label them as having mental health problems themselves. For example, the ward sister commented:

> (Overinvolvement has) never been a problem for me – but I've seen it with other nurses – it's usually the vulnerable ones with problems of their own who identify with patients – and it's usually the neurotic or manipulative patients they get involved with – if I ever see that happening I usually have a word with them for their own good ...

As a result of repeated disappointments when patients failed to improve and strong normative sanctions against overinvolvement or innovation, many nurses did withdraw from patients. However, as the comments of several nurses indicated, this process had its own costs and could lead to both a negative self-concept and a decreased capacity to relate to key individuals in the nurse's private life. The long-term effects which such actions could have on personal relationships and self-esteem were described by a male nurse:

> After a busy day or when patients have been playing up I tend to go home very tense – and my wife's just had a miscarriage and she's very depressed just now – and it tends to be 'Oh God, no, I've heard all this before'. I feel I've just come home from

work and it's starting over again as soon as I walk through the door – and the guilt adds to my stress really because if I've got time for anyone it should be my wife but the last thing you want when you go home is somebody hammering at you again. I do worry about it really because my first wife was a nurse up here too and I think a good 70% of our problem was that we turned off from each other's problems because of the work up here.

In conclusion, the interview data suggested that the nurses on this ward had a partial realization of the discrepancies between the official ideology of mental health nursing and the practical knowledge they used to organize their everyday activities within the ward situation. This knowledge often made them feel uncomfortable and could trigger attempts to alter their daily pattern of work activities. However, as the nurses' insights tended to form a piecemeal and individualized critique of discrete problems of organizational structure, patient characteristics and nursing action, rather than a coherent analysis of the whole range of factors influencing ward life, their attempts to improve the quality of care tended to underestimate the structural inter-relationships between various problems and to have a highly individualistic orientation. As a result, their attempts to help patients were often unsuccessful, which caused particular stress for those nurses who genuinely cared about patients and sought their main job satisfaction through helping them.

One solution to these feelings was to adopt a more instrumental attitude towards work. This attitude tended to be reinforced by the more highly qualified and experienced staff on the ward, who cautioned the more idealistic staff about overinvolvement with patients and the impracticality of changing the ward environment. The potential for change which was inherent in the nurses' partial understanding of, and dissatisfaction with, the problems of their working environment thus became channelled into the maintenance of the existing patterns of interaction and facilitated the recreation of the very system many nurses found dissatisfying and stress producing.

THE COMMUNITY UNIT

Introduction

The next section seeks to examine the work environment and perceptions of the community nurses and highlight the similarities and differences between the stresses that nurses experience within the ward and community settings. As this section will show, many community nurses enter this branch of the profession in the hope of escaping the stresses of life within the institution only to re-experience the process of disillusionment as life within the community fails to meet their initial expectation of a radical alternative to institutional care.

General description

The community unit at the research hospital was staffed by 14 nurses. In contrast to the ward all staff were fully qualified RMNs and around half had taken a one year postqualification course in community psychiatric nursing. The nurses each carried individual caseloads of approximately 35 patients, most of whom had been receiving treatment for about two years. As on the ward, around two thirds of the patients were female and a substantial proportion had been re-referred to the community nurses on several occasions and had lengthy histories of involvement with the psychiatric services. Whilst the community unit was theoretically intended to help prevent the 'revolving door syndrome' on the wards by providing follow-up care for patients discharged from the ward this seldom occurred in practice and the unit dealt with a distinct subgroup of patients whose involvement with psychiatry generally remained on an outpatient basis.

In contrast to the ward, where the nurses had collective responsibility for dealing with a group of patients within a ward environment dominated by the ethos of organic psychiatry and the need to maintain order, the community nurses were heavily committed to the ideal of establishing a personal relationship with their patients and helping them to resolve their problems through individual psychological counselling. The nurses saw their capacity to provide patients with individual attention through weekly or fortnightly home visits as a prime difference between the two settings and regarded the increased opportunities for patient contact provided by the community structure as an important source of both additional job satisfaction and stress.

The nurses' diaries

An excerpt from the diary of one of the community nurses (Figure 4.2) illustrates the way in which the social role of the mental health system in modern society ensured that the contradictions and stresses which often led the ward nurses to withdraw from patient contact were recreated within the community setting, despite the nurses' commitment to psychological rather than organic models of intervention.

The patient described in this excerpt was typical of many patients seen by the community nurses. She was a married woman in her early 50s with two adult children and a husband who was away from home

Nurses description of events	Nurse's comments
Telephone call from distressed client. Wants to see CPN today urgently.	Not my client but well known to all of us. Will have to visit as client not calmed on phone - but disrupts plans for today
Emergency visit to above client.	Irritated by this lady as did not listen to attempts to educate her about anxiety management. Has received many types of treatment from doctors, CPNs, etc. I feel she enjoys her problems.
	Unable to get away - client talks non-stop - seems to feel we have all day to spend with her.

Figure 4.2 Diary excerpt of a community nurse.

two or three nights a week on average. She had a history of agora-phobic and hypochondriacal symptoms and panic attacks extending back approximately 11 years. During this time she had been seen by a variety of health service professionals such as psychiatrists, psychologists and community psychiatric nurses and had a history of slight improvement followed by relapses whenever help was withdrawn. She was on tranquillizers which she tended to misuse by taking additional tablets whenever she felt agitated.

The patient's latest referral to the psychiatric community nursing service had occurred approximately six months previously and had been triggered by the fact that she was visiting her GP on a daily basis complaining of a variety of physical symptoms. Since being referred to the service her visits to the GP had declined to approximately one a week and had been replaced by an increasing reliance on the community nurses. She telephoned the nursing office several mornings a week demanding immediate home visits because she was no longer able to cope. If the nurses attempted to postpone their visits for more than a few hours the patient would retaliate by telephoning her GP or visiting the surgery in a hysterical state. As a lower status employee the nurse was therefore under two sets of obligations to continue seeing the patient and was susceptible to pressure from both the GP and the patient.

In order to avoid jeopardizing their relationship with her GP the nurses therefore tended to unofficially share this patient out amongst themselves and whoever was currently available either spent a lengthy telephone session reassuring her or made an emergency visit. The patient generally calmed down after these interventions and usually thanked the nurses profusely for the help they had just given her. This response seemed to engender ambivalent feelings in the staff who regarded her as both a problem patient with little real desire to improve and as someone whom they helped to stabilize and maintain in the community by visiting regularly. Thus, structural contradictions centring on the problem of patient versus professional responsibility locked this patient and the nurses into a pattern of repeated crisis orientated interactions which had similarities with many of the situations on the ward.

Interview data

The interview data revealed that the similarities in the interaction patterns between nurses and patients on the ward and in the community were a source of grave disappointment to many nurses and showed that for many nurses the pattern of an initially high level of commitment followed by increasing disillusionment and withdrawal was repeated within the community setting. In contrast to some critics of psychiatry who dismiss the move into the community as a mere change in location (Brown, 1985; Cohen, 1985; Scull, 1977), the community nurses were unanimous in perceiving community care as fundamentally different from institutional provision. Their reasons for believing this were based not only on the criteria they used for evaluating the institution but also on the personal meaning which changes in psychiatric practices held for them. From this perspective, there were significant differences between the ward and community settings as psychotropic medication was used less routinely and the nurses spent more time trying to understand the personal meaning of their patients' problems.

One of the most graphic illustrations of the personal impact of the changes which have taken place within psychiatry was provided by a nurse who had worked intermittently within the research hospital for over 30 years. Her testimony not only illustrates the magnitude of the changes which had taken place within the research hospital but also reveals how the community nurses' failure to perceive the underlying continuities within the structure of the mental health system could cause them to respond to changes in their work with initial enthusiasm followed by growing disillusionment, a response pattern which mirrored the sequence disclosed within the ward setting. The nurse described conditions within the hospital at the start of her career in the following terms:

> When I started here in the forties it was the old institution where all the doors were locked, knives and forks counted and locked away after meals, where there was no private clothing

at all – it was literally the era of the ticking shift and mass baths. When I came back I was amazed at the changes and it took me about six months to adjust to the fact that doors were now open and that people were wearing their own clothes, that where previously I'd worked on a ward where we had 100 beds in a massive dormitory there were now only 30 beds on a ward. I felt very insecure at first because previously it had been the old institution where the nurses walked about like prison warders with big bunches of keys hanging from their belts. I liked it eventually – I felt it was much better for patients and staff – but at first it made me feel very odd.

Although this nurse felt that conditions within the institution had changed dramatically during her absence she still became disillusioned with institutional work and eventully sought to escape from it:

Before I came here I spent three years on a long-stay ward and at the end of that I'd become institutionalized myself – I knew I just went in and did what I had to do routinely. It had got difficult to care any more and that made me feel quite bad about myself so I gave my notice in but the matron suggested I went into the community instead and when I did I thought, this is for me – challenge, responsibility, a chance to use my own initiative. I felt as though my work had some meaning again.

Whilst this nurse still regarded community work as radically different from ward nursing she revealed at a later stage in her interview that she was now experiencing many of the negative emotions which had led the ward based nurses to reject patient contact:

I often find I want to pull away from the client. This year at times I've been listening to clients and experiencing anxiety symptoms myself when a little voice inside me has been saying 'I must get out' and it's not specifically that I've got to get on to the next patient – it's just that the general stress has been so much that I need time to myself and I feel a need to get away. They don't have this on the wards; if the going gets too heavy you can always make an excuse – you know, 'I've got to put the linen away and give out the medication'. We have no way of escaping . . . and sometimes if I've put a lot of effort in and they demand more and more then it begins to feel like 'You're taking my blood' and it's not good to get into that position where you feel you've given someone a pound of flesh because you really find it very difficult to go on working with them.

The community nurses' feelings of resentment towards their patients were often compounded and complicated by their strong sense of personal responsibility for their patients. Such feelings were augmented by the individualized nature of the nurses' relationships with each of the patients in their particular caseload. All the nurses mentioned that their initial training had inculcated an almost parental sense of responsibility for their patients which could make it difficult for them to accept that patients had to take some responsibility for their own lives. As one nurse explained:

It's very hard for nurses to say that patients have to take responsibility for themselves. I think it stems back to the old idea that the nurse is someone who cares and who does things for people – and patients have expectations of you – they expect you to solve their problems and they find it hard to accept that sometimes you just can't.

The nurses' feelings of overwhelming personal responsibility for solving their patients' problems were compounded by doubts concerning their therapeutic competence and ability to cope effectively with a generic caseload. As a male nurse explained:

I think we're a jack of all trades and master of none. Many times we're afraid to say we can't help patients because we feel we've got to prove ourselves as a profession. I've got several cases at the moment that I'm taking without feeling very happy about the referral but I don't feel I can say I'm not expert enough to deal with that and just leave them – I feel any help is better than no help at all.

The nurses' desire to prove their worth as mental health professionals thus made it difficult for them to admit openly either that they were unable to perceive the solutions to the patients' problems or that the solutions lay in improved social conditions rather than psychiatric intervention. A major stratagem which they used to counter the insecurities generated by this problem involved moving away from their individual responsibilities for patients and attempting to recreate the collective responsibility of the ward situation by responding rapidly to putative emergencies and arranging with colleagues to provide additional back-up for difficult cases. Whilst this strategy helped alleviate their anxiety by giving them a greater degree of familiarity with their patients' problems and increasing the predictability of their working environment it also had the paradoxical effect of concomitantly increasing their doubts about their own competence by raising the possibility that their colleagues would be critical of their handling of a particular case and by escalating many of the problems between them and their patients. This meant that the nurses' attempts to solve the various problems they faced often had a similar outcome to those of the ward based nurses and helped perpetuate the various problems of the mental health system.

CONCLUSION

This chapter sets out to examine the effects which the organizational structure and ideology of the mental health system have on the daily actions and subjective experiences of mental health nurses and their patients. In contrast to most previous studies within the stress literature, which have implicitly assumed that we do not need detailed analyses of social structures in order to understand individual experience, this chapter has emphasized the reciprocal interplay between the structural and ideological features of a given social environment and the knowledge and activities of the various participants within it.

The three key problems described within the critical psychiatry literature were clearly apparent within the nurses' relationships with patients. The overt social control function of the mental health system was most obvious within the ward setting and was characterized by activities such as the control of patients who had been committed under section and the use of medication to subdue disruptive individuals. The more overt social control functions of their work were often recognized by the nurses and were frequently disliked by them as such activities tended to conflict with their self-image as helpers. In order to reduce the discrepancy between the two activities the nurses utilized various rationalizations which enabled them to reframe such activities as either legitimate sanctions directed at rational, but morally reprehensible individuals, who were abusing the mental health services and who were therefore undeserving of sympathy, or as therapeutic activities designed to help irrational individuals who were morally blameless, but who had forfeited their right to self-determination because of their mental illnesses. The therapeutic terminology of psychiatry was particularly important in legitimating the latter perspective as it enabled socially unacceptable behaviour to be reconceptualized as mental illness and its control interpreted as treatment, thus integrating the social control and treatment concerns of staff within a framework which maintained the concept of uncoercive care.

The clinical terminology of psychiatry therefore seemed to function not only as the expression of a shared organizational perspective but also as a mechanism through which the nurses could acquire a degree of emotional immunity from the more overt contradictions of the mental health system.

In addition to identifying the overt social control function of the mental health system, the critical psychiatry literature argues that the institution fulfils a more pervasive, covert or 'soft' social control function by promulgating individualistic explanations and treatment strategies which obscure the social implications of many patients' problems. This form of social control operated not only through the models which the nurses used to interpret their patients' problems but also through forms of work organization which segregated patients from one another. The nurses' desire to segregate patients was particularly apparent within the ward setting where the physical structure of the unit placed patients in close proximity with one another and sometimes led to the formation of social and emotional links between patients. The nurses generally regarded such relationships with suspicion and saw the development of group solidarity amongst patients as a highly stress provoking potential threat to their authority. In order to deal with such threats they tended to categorize group leaders as rational 'trouble makers' who should be excluded from the ward and to see other attachments as self-evidently pathological because they occurred between disturbed individuals. This enabled them to rationalize their attempts to undermine such relationships as being in the patients' best interests. Although the nurses tended to discourage relationships between patients they were equally suspicious of social isolates and patients who had difficulty coexisting amicably with their wardmates, fearing unpredictable outbursts of violence from such patients. From the nurses' point of view the ideal relationship between patients seemed to be one in which patients co-existed peaceably and communicated with each other in a distant and superficial manner.

The strategies which the nurses used to contain their anxieties about patients thus had the effect of fragmenting the group context of the ward and ensuring that the proximity of other individuals in similar circumstances became a mechanism for reaffirming the solitary nature of each patient's transactions with psychiatry rather than an opportunity for developing shared understanding and mutual support.

The individualized nature of the nurses' relationships with patients was equally evident within the community setting where the nurses each carried their own caseloads and interacted with each patient within a series of isolated relationships. Whilst the nurses were aware that many of their patients had similar problems and that these problems often centred around social isolation and feelings of intense loneliness and personal inadequacy, they were reluctant to bring their patients into contact with one another in order to explore such problems and offered a variety of reasons for this ranging from lack of suitable accommodation to the probability of medical opposition. Such problems certainly existed but rarely appeared insurmountable and more fundamental reasons seemed to be, firstly, that the nurses' immersion within the individualistic models of psychiatry meant that in practice they seldom paid much attention to the value of bringing patients together and secondly, that the prospect of group solidarity between patients was quite threatening for the nurses as it raised the possibility that their authority and therapeutic expertise would be challenged by the group. The nurses' own insecurities, which derived in part from the social isolation of their own work organization, thus contributed to the maintenance of interaction patterns which perpetuated the covert social control function of the mental health system by obscuring both the social implications of patients' problems and the possibility of socialized solutions.

The second major problem identified within the critical psychiatry literature centres on the idea that psychiatry is simultaneously committed to the alleviation of mental illness and to identifying increasingly subtle forms of behavioural deviation and personal distress as problems needing the expert intervention of trained mental health professionals. This paradox was particularly evident within the community setting where the nurses often seemed to regard the whole community as potential clients, a perception which resulted in a curious amalgamation between therapeutic imperialism and a siege mentality in their attitude towards their work. On the one hand, the nurses believed quite genuinely that people would benefit both from easier access to therapeutic help whilst their emotional problems were still relatively minor and from preventative exposure to psychiatric precepts before they developed problems. On the other hand, the nurses' perception that the whole community consisted of potential clients was extremely anxiety provoking for them as they felt that the demands on them were potentially limitless and that their workload could easily escalate beyond all control. As a result of this perception the nurses tended to avoid direct contact with the communities in which they worked and utilized the medical profession as gatekeepers who limited the number of referrals they received. Whilst this strategy helped to contain the nurses' anxieties concerning the potential size of their caseloads it also had the effect of reinforcing their tendency to equate community care with the care of individuals within the community and exacerbating their neglect of the communal aspects of their patients' problems.

The third problem identified within the critical psychiatry literature centres on the equivocal implications of psychiatric intervention for personal responsibility. Within this research one of the most striking features of nurse–patient relationships within both the ward and community settings was the degree of ambivalence which both parties revealed towards the asymmetries of responsibility and dependence which characterized their interactions. For the nurses, the perfect mental health patient was very similar to the ideal patient of general medicine and was someone who coped with their problems without constantly demanding help, but who was co-operative and grateful for any help given and who showed a capacity for insight and the ability to make constructive changes in their life as a result of the advice the nurses provided. Unfortunately for the nurses, their patients were, almost by definition, unlikely to conform to their ideal and as a result the nurses often bcame disillusioned and developed a more cynical view of patients as both manipulative and irresponsible. This perception could be disturbing for the more committed nurses as it conflicted with their own desired self-image as dedicated helpers.

The empirical data presented in this research thus suggests that the structural contradictions of the mental health system were reflected in the equivocal motives and understandings which the various participants habitually brought to their everyday interactions. As a result of these ambiguities, the activities of all parties tended to take place within various unacknowledged conditions and to have a range of unintended and paradoxical consequences. These could be highly distressing for all involved. Unfortunately, the structural problems which created the initial conditions for these unintended outcomes often ensured that the coping strategies which the various participants employed also rebounded upon them and had the unforeseen consequence of intensifying the initial tensions within the system. Thus, the conflicting strategies which the different participants employed to help them tackle the stresses facing them frequently interacted to help recreate many of the more pernicious aspects of organizational life and exacerbate the personal problems they were all attempting to resolve.

REFERENCES

Baron, C. (1987) *Asylum to Anarchy*, Free Association Books, London.

Baruch, G. and Treacher, A. (1978) *Psychiatry Observed*, Routledge and Kegan Paul, London.

Bott, E. (1976) Hospital and society. *British Journal of Medical Psychology*, **49**, 97–140.

Brown, P. (1985) *The Transfer of Care*, Routledge and Kegan Paul, London.

Busfield, J. (1986) *Managing Madness, Changing Ideas and Practice*, Hutchinson, London.

Castel, R., Castel, F. and Lovell, A. (1982) *The Psychiatric Society*, Columbia University Press, New York.

Cherniss, C. (1980) *Staff Burnout: Job Stress in the Human Services*, Sage, London.

Cohen, S. (1985) *Visions of Social Control*, Polity Press, Cambridge.

Conrad, P. and Schneider, J. (1980) *Deviance and Medicalization. From Badness to Sickness*, C.V. Mosby, London.

Eaton, W. (1986) *The Sociology of Mental Disorders*, Praeger, New York.

Goffman, E. (1971) *Asylums*, Penguin, Harmondsworth.

Handy, J. (1988) Theoretical and methodological problems within occupational stress and burnout research. *Human Relations*, **41**, 351–70.

Horowitz, A. (1982) *The Social Control of Mental Illness*, Academic Press, London.

Ingleby, D. (ed.) (1981) *Critical Psychiatry: The Politics of Mental Health*, Penguin, Harmondsworth.

Ingelby, D. (1985) Mental health and social order, in *Social Control and the State*, (eds S. Cohen and A. Scull), Basil Blackwell, Oxford.

Mangen, P. (1982) *Sociology and Mental Health*, Churchill Livingstone, Edinburgh.

Miller, P. and Rose, N. (eds) (1986) *The Power of Psychiatry*, Polity Press, Cambridge.

Morgan, D. (1975) Explaining mental illness. *Archives Europeenes de Sociologie*, **16**, 262–80.

Newton, T. (1989) Occupational stress and coping with stress: a critique. *Human Relations*, **42**, 441–61.

Payne, R. and Firth-Cozens, J. (Eds) (1987) *Stress in Health Professionals*, John Wiley and Sons, Chichester.

Penfold, S. and Walker, G. (1984) *Women and the Psychiatric Paradox*, Open University Press, Milton Keynes.

Pines, A. and Maslach, C. (1978) Characteristics of staff burnout in mental health settings. *Hospital and Community Psychiatry*, **29**, 233–7.

Ramon, S. (1985) *Psychiatry in Britain: Meaning and Policy*, Croom Helm, London.

Scheper-Hughes, N. and Lovell, A. (1986) Breaking the circuit of social control: lessons in public psychiatry from Italy and Franco Basaglia. *Social Science and Medicine*, **23**, 159–78.

Scheper-Hughes, N. and Lovell, A. (eds) (1987) *Psychiatry Inside Out: Selected Writings of Franco Basaglia*, Colombia University Press, New York.

Scott, R. (1973) The treatment barrier (Pts 1 and 2). *British Journal of Medical Psychology*, **46**, 45–67.

Scull, A. (1977) *Decarceration: Community Treatment and the Deviant*, Prentice-Hall, New Jersey.

Turner, B . (1987) *Medical Power and Social Knowledge*, Sage, London.

Wallis, D. and de Wolff, C. (eds) (1988) *Stress and Organizational Problems in Hospitals*, Croom Helm, London.

CHAPTER 5

The Claybury CPN Stress Study: background and methodology

Leonard Fagin and Heather Bartlett

BACKGROUND

Current health service reforms have set a seal of approval on efforts made by mental health professionals over the past four decades to focus care of individuals close to their communities and outside large institutions. Community psychiatric nurses (CPNs) have been at the forefront of this crusade. In his views to the House of Commons Select Committee on Social Services, the Director of the Hospital Advisory Service, Peter Horrocks, said:

> The CPN is probably the most important single professional in the process of moving the care of mental illness into the community.
> (House of Commons Social Services Committee, 1985)

This view has been supported by the marked increase in CPNs across the country (White, 1990) (Figure 5.1) and it is the mental health profession which has experienced the greatest growth. Most districts now possess thriving CPN departments, based either in hospitals or community mental health facilities. In North East Thames Region alone, CPN numbers have increased by 72.6% in the past five years. This rapid expansion, alongside changing roles and expectations, has imposed considerable pressures on a relatively young and developing professional group (Brooker, 1985; White, 1990).

Nobody would now doubt that community psychiatric nursing has an important part to play in the network of psychiatric services. It has a well-respected tradition of nearly 40 years, since 1954, when Lena Peat and Dr Rees (Peat and Watt, 1984) first took the courageous step of focusing aftercare of discharged psychiatric patients from

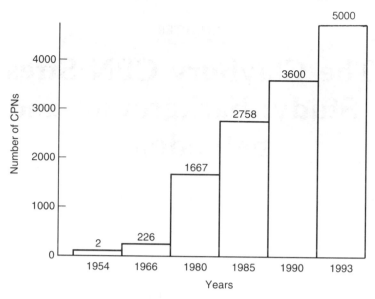

Figure 5.1 CPN growth 1954–1993.

Warlingham Park in their own homes and day centres in Croydon. At the time, these tentative moves to leave the psychiatric institution were considered radical and, to say the least, quite risky and few nurses were initially tempted to leave the protection of the asylum.

CPN work has been transfigured since then. Rapid changes have imposed considerable demands on CPN services, not only in terms of increasing the sometimes impossible caseloads but also by broadening their field of intervention far beyond the training of the traditional psychiatric nurse. Attachments to primary care teams have loosened their ties to multidisciplinary secondary mental health services, a move which has met with some criticism as CPNs are asked to deal with increasing numbers of depressed and neurotic patients without much supervision. There is concern that this has been done at the expense of the care of the chronic mentally ill patient (Goldberg, 1985).

In these settings CPNs enjoy more autonomy in decision making (Skidmore and Friend, 1985), but sometimes find themselves adrift when having to decide priorities arising from referrals from psychiatric teams. In these conditions, it does not come as a surprise to receive memoranda from CPN departments conveying their inability to deal with any more referrals or CPNs candidly saying that they are not enjoying their work as much as they used to. A Manpower Services report suggested that absenteeism in nursing had increased to an average of 14 days per year since the introduction of the health service market in the UK, especially amongst those who were concerned over excessive workloads (Seecombe and Buchan, 1993).

Current NHS reforms and hospital closures have added to these pressures, so much so that CPNs could become the first casualties of change. In our view, their determination to pioneer often singlehandedly new community services has put them in vulnerable positions, not only as a professional group but also because often they are asked to deal with impossible problems in an isolated manner.

The NHS does not have a good tradition when it comes to looking after its own personnel, especially in times when reforms seem to be guided by government and management according to the latest political whim or when planning appears to be financially driven rather than based on clinical advice and knowhow. It makes sense to ensure that those entrusted with the care of mentally disturbed persons are themselves emotionally supported in their work. We have all had personal experiences of mental health workers buckling under the strain and yet they are expected to know how to cope with their own difficulties and leave them aside when dealing with their clients' problems.

In summary, the intrinsic nature of the job is often inherently stressful, dealing with people at various extremes of emotional distress. If, in addition to this, we pour into the melting pot radical changes in financial and management structures, shifts of allegiance to primary care, nursing audit on levels and quality of performance, an increasing range of psychiatric disorders that require nursing intervention and, last but not least, uncertainties over employment futures, we can begin to appreciate current occupational pressures on the CPN role.

OCCUPATIONAL STRESS RESEARCH
IN HEALTH PROFESSIONS

Stress related to work in the health professions has only recently attracted the attention of investigators (Edelwich and Brodsky, 1980; Farber, 1983; Payne and Firth-Cozens, 1987). High levels of stress have been reported as contributing to staff burnout and have been described in health visitors (Goodwin, 1983; West *et al.*, 1988), district nurses (MacLellan, 1990), occupational therapists (Sweeney *et al.*, 1991; Rees and Smith, 1991), social workers (Bennett *et al.*, 1993), clinical psychology trainees (Cushway, 1992), medical students (Firth, 1986), senior house officers (Firth-Cozens, 1987), doctors (Mawardi, 1979) and junior psychiatrists in residency programmes (Russell *et al.*, 1975). Interestingly, psychiatrists seem so far to have escaped scrutiny, although anecdotal accounts suggest that this group of professionals is predictably as vulnerable as others to stress and burnout (Margison, 1987).

Stress levels in nursing appear to be on the increase, if a *Nursing Times* survey is to be believed (Cole, 1992). Although this was a self-selected sample of respondents to a questionnaire in a magazine, 1800 nurses took the time to reply; 93% of nurses said that they felt stressed at work and a quarter of the sample estimated that stress levels were 'very high'. Seventeen percent intended to leave the profession in the following year and 71% thought the problems in the National Health Service would worsen. Nurses ranked the major stressors, 65% pinpointing excessive workloads, 61% management related stress, 54% lack of resources and 49% changes in the NHS. Noticeable in these findings was the fact that the highest stressors were organizational and managerial, whilst patient related stressors were consistently at the bottom of the list. Nurses also reported physical and psychological stress related symptoms, including headaches, sleep problems, tiredness, moodiness and irritability, frustration, anxiety and poor concentration. A third of the sample said that stress was likely to make them accident-prone at work.

These findings seem to be confirmed in research into different aspects of general nursing carried out to date. Gray-Toft and Anderson (1981a, 1981b) reported on aspects of stress experienced in general nurses, after developing a nursing stress scale, scoring the frequency with which nurses found situations stressful. Examining responses in five different environments (medical-surgical, cardiovascular, surgical, oncology and hospice) stress emanated from three distinct sources: workload, inadequate preparation and dealing with death and dying issues.

Nichols *et al*. (1981) investigated stress by asking nurses to choose from predefined aspects of their work which could be considered stressful, with negative and positive connotations being assumed by researchers rather than their respondents. Cross and Fallon (1985) added to this the dimension of personal impact, comparing findings in different ward settings.

Dewe (1987), in a New Zealand sample of over 2000 respondents to a postal questionnaire, explored the relationship between frequency of demand, how the situation taxed the nurse in terms of tension experienced and the effects of stress in terms of tiredness. This aimed at dealing more comprehensively with the stressor–stress relationship, a fact which is often overlooked in stress research. Frequency of demand was not always associated with indicators of individual stress. For example, the regular and predictable difficulties associated with nursing the critically ill may be associated with tension and tiredness, but unrelenting work overload may ultimately be more damaging to personal health and job satisfaction. Dewe also identified the coping strategies used by nurses and, using component analysis, described six dimensions. These involved:

1. problem-orientated behaviours, such as rationalization and delegation;
2. unwinding strategies such as distraction, expression of feelings and frustration to colleagues;
3. keeping problems to oneself;
4. acceptance;
5. resignation;
6. avoidance behaviours, such as smoking, drinking tea, coffee and alcohol.

Unfortunately, none of these studies was complemented by face-to-face interviews or qualitative data.

Not all nursing environments are equally stressful. A number of investigations have identified coronary and intensive care units as particularly prone to high levels of stress (Vreeland and Ellis, 1969; Hay and Oken, 1972). Hipwell *et al.* (1989), investigating stress in four different ward environments in Birmingham, UK, found that dealing with death and dying issues was particularly stressful for nurses working in specialized units such as coronary care and renal units, whilst work overload was a major stressor for nurses in non-specialized medical and geriatric wards. Of interest was the finding that dissatisfaction with the work environment, especially if it differed markedly from perceived ideals as measured on the Work Environment Scale (Moos and Insel, 1981), was a good predictor of occupational stress. In Nebraska, similar findings were reported by Foxall *et al.* (1990). Although indicating that overall job stress was high, it was not significantly different in varied ward milieus; what changed was the quality of the specific stressor. This has obvious implications for specific stress management programmes.

To date there has been little published research on stress and the psychiatric nurse and only anecdotal accounts of the pressured working lives of CPNs have been described in nursing journals (Mendlson, 1993a, 1993b; McMahon, 1993). The following description sheds some light on the problems faced by CPNs in a typical day's work.

Jean Collins pulled into the car park at 9.20 a.m.; she was late because of the rush hour traffic and already behind schedule. Quickly checking her diary, she calculated that if she skipped lunch she could probably manage to catch up.

She left the office shortly afterwards to visit her first client, Michael Clarke, whose mother had died recently. This had upset Michael's mental state and it was important he received his medication and that his condition be monitored at least on a weekly basis.

Approaching the local authority owned tower block where Michael lived, Jean was too frightened to enter, as there was a small group of young men next to the lift. Back on the road, she struggled in London's usual heavy traffic.

After one home visit, Jean stopped to make a list of all the telephone calls she would need to make later at the office. The secretary was off sick and she would have to speak to each referring agency about their clients. No letters would be typed until the secretary recovered.

Later that day, Jean returned to the tower block. This time she had persuaded a male CPN colleague to accompany her. When they saw Michael it was clear that his mental state had deteriorated. His flat smelt, the dishes did not appear to have been washed since Jean's last visit and Michael had neglected his self-care.

Jean and her colleague agreed that Michael ought to see his GP or psychiatrist urgently so that an admission to hospital could be arranged. Walking to her car, Jean wondered what problems she might have in contacting these busy professionals late on a Friday afternoon.

(Carson *et al.*, 1993)

Many CPNs would relate to the above fictional account. Added to this they have to cope with the lack of community resources they can refer on to, waiting lists for day centres, permanently engaged telephones in GPs' surgeries and social services and never-ending traffic jams. Experiences of violence towards CPNs are far from uncommon and many will have this at the back of their minds when out on their visits.

Cronin-Stubbs and Brophy (1984) examined burnout in American psychiatric nurses and compared them with their colleagues in other nursing disciplines. Burnout was associated with more conflicts with patients, relatives and staff than in general nursing and psychiatric nurses also experienced less affirmation on the job, which Cronin-Stubbs and Brophy attributed to psychiatric interventions being less observable and outcomes less tangible than with intensive care nurses. They also concluded that psychiatric nurses tend to be less inter-dependent than surgical nurses and less able to separate their work from personal relationships at home. Their results suggested that psychiatric nurses were in need of extra emotional and practical support.

Earlier, Rump (1979) in Australia examined job satisfaction and hospital size, with satisfaction decreasing as hospital size increases. This study contradicts expectations of distress experienced by psychiatric nurses moving away from large institutions to smaller psychiatric units, where nurses have been described as having to overcome difficulties in adapting to deinstitutionalized environments.

Jones *et al*. (1987) from the Applied Psychology Unit at the University of Sheffield, examined psychological stress in special hospital nurses. Following Payne's occupational stress model (Payne, 1979), health and well-being were measured in relation to job demands, job constraints and supports as well as level of job satisfaction. They reported levels of psychological distress higher than expected in other employed samples (although not higher than unemployed cohorts), with females scoring higher than their male counterparts. Unsurprisingly in this context, health and well-being were strongly correlated with what the authors described as 'aversive' demands, where nurses were asked to undertake work which they considered unnecessary or work with patients they were afraid of. Job satisfaction was considered to be considerably lower than other employed samples, especially if their spouses were also working at the hospital, indicating the difficulty in separating work and home concerns.

In the Netherlands, Landeweerd and Boumans (1988) examined work satisfaction, health and stress in nurses working in an admissions ward, in two short-stay psychotherapeutic units and two long-stay units. Although the numbers in their sample were small, the short-stay unit experienced highest stress scores attributable to pressures to take in patients from the admissions ward, difficulties in transferring patients to other wards, dealing with patients with no positive prognosis and small amount of positive feedback from patients.

Psychiatric nurses formed a large proportion of the sample of nurses in Firth *et al*.'s (1987) investigation into burnout and support in long-stay nursing in Northumberland. They reported high levels of depersonalization in the Maslach Burnout Inventory scores in their sample, as well as higher levels of depression than in the general population, experience of emotional 'draining' and avoidance of decisions at work. These were influenced by the presence or lack of support from a professional 'superior' and role clarity at work, especially in describing what was expected from each nurse in the context of service philosophy and priorities.

Unfortunately, a number of methodological problems are apparent in current research into nursing stress literature. The small sample size and the specificity of the units investigated make generalizations difficult as far as the profession of nursing is concerned. This may indicate the need to look at specific stressors for specific types of nursing. With a few exceptions, the majority of studies fail to use properly constructed, reliable and validated measurement tools and much of the findings arise out of anecdotal accounts and often the results are contradictory and confusing (Power and Sharp, 1988).

Furthermore, there are no major studies looking at specific stressors for community psychiatric nurses. It is difficult to understand why this is the case, as CPNs have made a radical change in the traditional role of the psychiatric nurse and one where stress related work conditions have been anecdotally referred to in professional journals. Handy (1990) attempted to develop a sociocultural explanation of psychiatric nursing practice, focusing on wards as well as community psychiatric nursing. As a participant-observer she described interesting differences between acute and elderly CPN teams.

The Community Psychiatric Nursing Journal has recently dedicated a number of articles to the subject of stress and burnout, attesting to the fact that this is a major cause for concern for the profession (Grevatt, 1993; Schafer, 1992). Furthermore, few studies have taken into account associated factors which may have a bearing on the results, such as qualifications and nursing grade, duration of nursing experience, caseloads and quality and frequency of supervision, all of which could have a bearing on how stressed nurses respond to challenging demands. Added to this, few studies investigate stressors and coping behaviours, especially focusing on strategies which could inform managers and planners on how to reduce stress at work.

As an aside, there is a paucity of research looking at the effects of burnout on the quality of patient care. Although this poses considerable methodological problems, it strikes one as obvious that stressed nurses will perform their duties with considerable handicap and that this may affect substantially how patients respond to nursing interventions and ultimately their health (Meyer, 1962; Meyer and Mendelson, 1961).

STRESS AND BURNOUT

The philosopher Locke in 1690 acknowledged that 'though the faculties of the mind are improved by exercise, they must not be put to a stress beyond their strength'. In modern dictionaries definitions of stress describe the force or pressure exercised on persons for the purpose of compulsion or extortion, as well as the strained effort or exertion needed to fulfil particular tasks. More recently, researchers have found the word stress to be too vague and all-encompassing a concept (Rutter, 1981). Some question its very existence (Engel, 1985). For the purpose of our own study we have adopted the simple definition outlined by Atkinson (1988) of an 'excess of demands over the individual's ability to meet them'. This captures the dynamic and temporal elements of stress and sees it as a struggle between coping strategies and external 'real world' pressures which impinge on individuals and have subjective and sometimes physical consequences.

These different components of stress can be incorporated into a circular model (Figure 5.2) which includes situational or external demands,

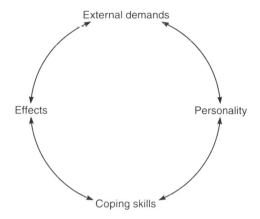

Figure 5.2 A stress model (adapted from Cooper *et al.*, 1988).

individual personality characteristics, coping strategies and subjective and physical consequences, which in turn influence the external environment.

External demands

The external demands are sometimes confused with the causes of stress, but must not be seen as indicating straightforward causality. Causes are often determined by the interaction of the different components. The external factors include intrinsic features (what people actually do) as well as extrinsic aspects of the job (management structures, performance goals, pay and conditions of service, peer relationships, etc.). As can be seen from this model, stress is not usually determined by single pressures but a complex mixture of forces with different weightings. To this must be added the temporal dimension. Stressors may occur suddenly and unexpectedly, as in radical changes of management structures, translocations, unanticipated absenteeism, or gradually and cumulatively, as in increasing caseloads, deterioration of peer relationships, inappropriate surroundings.

Personality characteristics

Personality features affect the way in which stressors are managed and subjectively experienced. People have low or high thresholds when coping with extra pressures and this is often determined by personal background and previous acquaintance with challenging situations. These features are closely linked with those aspects of personality that increase or decrease self-confidence and self-esteem. Clearly, success in managing previous stressors increases thresholds to the perception of future threatening events and allows some professionals to take extra difficulties in their stride. Others will feel that even small additions to demands will be experienced as major problems, making proverbial mountains out of molehills. Firth *et al.* (1987), for example, noted that those suffering from burnout tended to direct anger towards themselves and avoid problems or decisions. Conversely, those that only directed anger onto others would report more difficulties in relating to patients and have negative views about them.

Coping strategies

Over time professionals increase their armamentarium of coping skills, gained mostly through trial and error as they face novel situations. Some professionals are likely to benefit from the support and guidance of more experienced staff, in the context of joint working or super-vision, whilst others predominantly learn on the job, adding new skills as they go along. Difficulties sometimes emerge when professionals use their acquired skills rigidly, without making the necessary adap-tations to variations in type or quality of demand. Some of the coping skills may address the problem in hand, but may have unfortunate consequences elsewhere. For example, an appropriate decision to work jointly with potentially violent patients in isolated tenement blocks may reduce the ability of the CPN team to respond to extra referrals, increasing waiting lists and putting more pressure on the service.

Once again, it is important to bear in mind that it is rare to find a coping response that doesn't have an impact on other aspects of the work. Some coping skills, however, are clearly maladaptive and it is therefore dubious to classify them as coping behaviours. Avoidance responses, for example in the shape of increasing absenteeism, may deal with anxieties in the short term but clearly impose further problems in the future.

Consequences of stress

The effects of stress can be detected in three distinct areas. **Subjec-tive experiences** include anxiety, depression, constant worry and para-doxical emotional detachment. These may be acknowledged or denied, often perceived by those around rather than by the person themselves. **Physical consequences** comprise the whole gamut of psychosomatic disturbances from the relatively trivial, such as short lived migraines or skin rashes, through the moderate and discomforting, such as irritable bowel syndrome and back problems, to the life-threatening disorders such as heart conditions and cerebrovascular accidents. **Behavioural changes** range from minor irritability to irascibility, resorting to addictive habits, alcoholism and smoking, or other avoidance behaviours such as the need to constantly change jobs, reluctance to take on further tasks or constant querulous relationships with managers and employers.

We can now move on to describe the **burnout stress syndrome** (Cherniss, 1980; Maslach, 1982) characterized by a triad of features:

1. **Exhaustion**: loss of energy; increase of distrust and cynicism; lowering of coping threshold making it increasingly more difficult to cope with extra, even trivial, commitments; difficulties in personal relationships; negative expectations with associated ruminations on failure rather than success.
2. **Depression**: hopelessness; loss of self-esteem and confidence.
3. **Psychosomatic troubles and addictive behaviour**.

THE CLAYBURY CPN STRESS STUDY

In an earlier study, we investigated the effects of unemployment on individuals and their families (Fagin, 1985). Whilst undertaking this research, it soon became obvious to us that work, as well as unemployment, could be damaging to health. This drew us to investigate the effects of mental health work on those that were given the responsibility to deliver it It struck us that clinicians' health was being taken for granted and yet we could see the emotional and sometimes physical effects of stress all around us in our working environment. this not only affected interpersonal relationships within working teams, but also the style of health care delivery, although this was rarely acknowledged.

Few staff were prepared to share with others how they were personally affected by the work they were undertaking or disclose their own limitations. In health care it is difficult for workers to say 'No, we can't manage within our present resources, whether personal or material'.

The pilot study

In a pilot investigation which preceded our study, Carson and his colleagues (1991, 1993) conducted the first published study looking at stress in CPNs. This study in turn led to the development of a CPN Stress Questionnaire, specifically aimed at addressing particular stressors for CPNs. To do this they conducted open-ended interviews with 16 CPNs in four districts. Respondents were asked what they found stressful about their work and they transcribed their responses. From these interviews, they were able to construct a questionnaire with 66 items, later reduced to 48.

The findings from this study, administering questionnaires to 61 CPNs in four NETRHA districts, revealed some unexpected results. For example, in two of the four districts, 'interruptions in the office' and 'trying to keep up a good quality of care in my work' were considered to be the most stressful responses. The working environment was also mentioned as highly stressful, as in 'having to visit unsafe areas'. More predictably, some clinical issues were also rated highly as top stressors. These included 'having to deal with suicidal clients on my own'. They also noted items which had low scores. These included being supported by colleagues, having enough contact with each other and describing internal communication and supervision within the team as causing no extra stress. More worryingly, CPNs were scoring high on the GHQ-28, a measure to ascertain the probability of pscyhiatric problems requiring specialized help. These figures were at least double those observed in ward based psychiatric nurses. CPNs were also recording low levels of job satisfaction and attributing their stress to the isolated nature of their work and taking on more responsibilities than ward based nurses.

The researchers were aware that although CPNs might be working in highly stressful situations, this did not necessarily imply that they were affected by them. They may have developed good personal coping strategies or alternatively, good support networks. To discover what coping strategies CPNs were using, a further 21 individual interviews were conducted with CPNs in the same four districts originally surveyed; 81% of the sample reported that the best strategy was to discuss their problems with colleagues. The most popular coping behaviour (24%) was either to smoke or have a coffee break; 19% sought relaxation in alternative tasks, such as listening to music or going out for a walk. Overall, however, the researchers noted a narrow range of coping strategies in the sample. When asked what suggestions they could offer their managers to reduce stress, 33% put forward a reduction in their caseload and 24% proposed employing more staff, having more supervision, in-service education and changes in managerial style (giving staff more praise).

The main study

The findings from the pilot study stimulated the researchers to undertake a more ambitious project. The Claybury CPN Stress Study was to be the largest study of its kind ever undertaken in the United Kingdom. A locally organised research scheme grant was obtained from the North East Thames Regional Health Authority to interview

CPNs working in the 16 districts of the NETRHA, a total of 250 CPNs. Only one of the districts did not participate in the study. A comparison group of 323 ward based psychiatric nurses was obtained from seven psychiatric units in the same region, either in large psychiatric hospitals or DGH units, taking in nurses from acute inpatient settings and continuing care wards.

In contrast to previous research into nursing stress, the researchers undertook to obtain a large sample of respondents which would allow a more reliable analysis of data. Validated measurement instruments were selected so that data could be compared with previous research into job stress. To understand stress in a more integrated model, coping behaviours were also analysed. The study also utilized qualitative data information to address specific issues not picked up by the measurement tools, such as the importance of group discussions and suggestions for improvements in CPN teams.

The original hypothesis arose from Carson *et al.*'s pilot study and predicted that CPNs would show more evidence of stress than ward based psychiatric nurses.

The objectives of the study were as follows:

1. To examine the variety, frequency and severity of stressors amongst CPNs in the NETRHA.
2. To describe coping strategies used by CPNs to reduce levels of occupational stress.
3. To compare occupational stress in CPNs with ward based psychiatric nurses, matched for age, sex and experience.
4. To provide feedback on the study's findings to all individuals and districts participating in the study.
5. To provide recommendations to CPNs and their managers on work stressors and effective coping strategies.
6. To disseminate the findings of the study to a wider audience.

Materials and methods

In this study, both quantitative and qualitative methods were used to investigate stress and coping in psychiatric nurses.

Quantitative indicators

These were administered to all CPNs and ward based staff. The tools used were especially selected to discover specific features contributing to occupational stress along the model described above. As will be seen, some measuring devices were able to focus on one or more stages of the stress pathway, for example, giving information on both stressors and effects.

1. **Demographic details**. This information gave indicators of personal experience, such as age, length of professional experience and time in current post, qualifications, client caseload, job security, support from line manager, quality and frequency of supervision.

2. **General Health Questionnaire (GHQ-28) (Goldberg and Williams, 1988)**. This well-validated 28-item inventory examines the symptoms of stress and indicates probability of psychiatric breakdown. A score of five or more items indicates 'psychiatric caseness'.

3. **Maslach Burnout Inventory (Maslach and Jackson, 1986)**. This tool looks at the long-term effects of stress in terms of emotional exhaustion, depersonalization (or distancing from personal relationships) and personal accomplishment. Scores can be classified according to low, moderate or high levels of burnout.

4. **Rosenberg Self-Attitude Questionnaire (Rosenberg, 1965)**. This gives an indication of self-esteem. Scores range between 10 and 40, the lower scores indicating higher self-opinion.

5. **Minnesota Job Satisfaction Scale (Koelbel *et al.*, 1991)**. This scale was specially designed to measure levels of job satisfaction for nurses. Higher scores indicate higher job satisfaction.

6. **Coping Skills Questionnaire (Cooper *et al.*, 1988)**. Looking at strategies used to deal with occupational stress. This scale was devised for British business managers. The strategies explored include social support, organization of tasks, logical approaches to stress, home and work relationships, awareness and management of time and involvement in or identification with work aims. The higher the score, the higher the number of strategies used to deal with stress related situations.

7. **Claybury CPN Stress Questionnaire (Carson *et al.*, 1993)**. This previously described self-administered questionnaire comprises 48 items on which subjects are asked to score on a 5-point scale, from '0 = This causes me no stress' to '4 = This causes me extreme stress'. This was the only questionnaire which was not administered to ward based staff as it is specific to CPNs.

Qualitative methodology

After each CPN department was surveyed a randomly selected subsample of approximately 20% of total CPNs was included in the qualitative phase of the research. This comprised two separate data gathering opportunities.

1. One-to-one interviews. A semistructured interview, focusing on personal issues of stress and coping.

2. Group discussions. These taped discussions followed an agenda set by the researcher, but allowed freeflowing discussion among a group of CPNs from the same department.

Statistical analysis

These used a range of available procedures, including parametric, non-parametric and multivariate techniques. Thanks to the large sample size, comparisons and correlations were possible both between and within samples of CPNs and ward based nurses. These included standard and multiple analysis of variance, analysis of covarying variables and an examination of regressional patterns to explore the possibility of predictive dimensions of stress and coping.

The following chapters will describe the main quantitative and qualitative findings from our study, as well as the implications and recommendations arising from them. We are indebted to all the CPNs who participated so enthusiastically and we hope we have been able to do justice to their insights and comments. Their willingness to be candid about their difficulties at work made our own efforts all the easier and more worthwhile and, by the publication of our research, we also hope that in small measure we may be contributing to the betterment of a valued profession.

REFERENCES

Atkinson, J. (1988) *Coping with Stress at Work*, Thorsons, Wellingborough.

Bennett, P., Evans, R. and Tattersall, A. (1993) Stress and coping in social workers: a preliminary investigation. *British Journal of Social Work*, **23**, 31–44.

Brooker, C. (1985) The 1985 National Community Psychiatric Nursing Survey Update: implications of the findings for the evolution of a survey methodology. Unpublished MSc thesis, City University. Quoted in Simmons, S. and Brooker, D. (1986) *Community Psychiatric Nursing. A Social Perspective*, Heinemann, London.

Carson, J., Bartlett, H. and Croucher, P. (1991) Stress in community psychiatric nursing: a preliminary investigation. *Community Psychiatric Nursing Journal*, **11**(2), 8–12.

Carson, J., Bartlett, H., Leary, J., Gallagher, T., Senapati-Sharma, M. (1993) Stress and the CPN. *Nursing Times*, **89**(3), 38–40.

Cherniss, C. (1980) *Professional Burnout in Human Service Organisations*, Praeger, New York.

Cole, A. (1992) High Anxiety. *Nursing Times*, **88**(12), 26–30.

Cooper, C., Sloan, S.J. and Williams, S. (1988) *Occupational Stress Indicator Management Guide*, NFER-Nelson, Windsor.

Cronin-Stubbs, D. and Brophy, E.B. (1984) Burnout: can social support save the psychiatric nurse? *Journal of Psychosocial Nursing in Mental Health Services*, **23**, 8–13.

Cross, D.G. and Fallon, A. (1985) A stressor comparison of four specialty areas. *Australian Journal of Advanced Nursing*, **13**, 43–5.

Cushway, D. (1992) Stress in clinical psychology trainees. *British Journal of Clinical Psychology*, **31**, 169–79.

Dewe, J. (1987) Identifying strategies nurses use to cope with stress. *Journal of Advanced Nursing*, **12**, 489–97.

Edelwich, J. and Brodsky, A. (1980) *Burnout: States of Disillusionment in the Helping Professions*, Human Sciences Press, New York.

Engel, B.T. (1985) Stress is a noun, no, a verb, no, an adjective, in *Stress and Coping*, (eds T.M. Field, P. McCabe and N. Schneidermann), Hillsdale, New York.

Fagin, L. (1985) Stress and unemployment. *Journal of Stress Medicine*, **1**, 27–36.

Farber, B.A. (1983) *Stress and Burnout in the Human Service Professions*, Pergamon, New York.

Firth, H., McKeown, P., McIntee, J. and Britton, P. (1987) Burnout, personality and support in long-stay nursing. *Nursing Times*, **83**(32), 55–7.

Firth, J. (1986) Levels and sources of stress in medical students. *British Medical Journal*, **292**, 1177–80.

Firth-Cozens, J. (1987) Emotional distress in junior house officers. *British Medical Journal*, **295**, 533–6.

Foxall, M.J., Zimmerman, L., Standley, R. and Bene, B. (1990) A comparison of frequency and sources of nursing job stress perceived by intensive care, hospice and medical-surgical nurses. *Journal of Advanced Nursing*, **15**, 577–84.

Goldberg, D. (1985) *Implementation of Mental Health Policies in Lancashire*. Paper presented at a joint DHSS/Royal College of Psychiatrists Conference on Community Care, London.

Goldberg, D. and Williams, P. (1988) *A User's Guide to the General Health Questionnaire*, NFER-Nelson, Windsor.

Goodwin, S. (1983) The stresses of health visiting. *Health Visitor*, **56**(1), 20–1.

Grevatt, H. (1993) Avoiding burnout. *Community Psychiatric Nursing Journal*, **13**(5), 6–9.

Gray-Toft, P. and Anderson, J. (1981a) The nursing stress scale: development of an instrument. *Journal of Behavioural Assessment*, **3**, 11–23.

Gray-Toft, P. and Anderson, J. (1981b) Stress amongst hospital nursing staff: its causes and effects. *Social Science and Medicine*, **15**, 639–47.

Handy, J. (1990) *Occupational Stress in a Caring Profession*, Gower, Aldershot.

Hay, D. and Oken, D. (1972) The psychological stresses of intensive care unit nursing. *Psychosomatic Medicine*, **34**, 109–18.

Hipwell, A.E., Tyler, P.A. and Wilson, C.M. (1989) Sources of stress and dissatisfaction among nurses in four hospital environments. *British Journal of Medical Psychology*, **62**, 71–9.

House of Commons Social Services Committee (1985) *Community Care with Special Reference to the Adult Mentally Ill and Mentally Handicapped People*, Second Report From the Social Services Committee, Session 1984–5, Chair: Mrs R. Short. HMSO, London.

Jones, J., Janman, K., Payne, R. *et al.* (1987) Some determinants of stress in psychiatric nurses. *International Journal of Nursing Studies*, **24**(2), 129–44.

Koelbel, P., Fuller, F. and Misener, T. (1991) Job satisfaction of nurse practitioners: an analysis using Herzberg's theory. *Nurse Practitioner*, **16**(4), 43–6.

Landeweerd, J. and Boumans, M. (1988) Nurses' work satisfaction and feelings of health and stress in three psychiatric departments. *International Journal of Nursing Studies*, **25**(3), 225–340.

MacLellan, M. (1990) Burnout in district nurses. *Journal of District Nursing*, February, 14–18.

Margison, F. (1987) Stress in Psychiatrists, in *Stress in Health Professionals*, (eds R. Payne and J. Firth-Cozens), John Wiley and Sons, Chichester.

Maslach, C. (1982) *Burnout: The Cost of Caring*, Prentice-Hall, New York.

Maslach, C. and Jackson, S. (1986) *Maslach Burnout Inventory*, Consulting Psychologists Press, California.

Mawardi, B.H. (1979) Satisfactions, dissatisfactions, and causes of stress in medical practice. *Journal of the American Medical Association*, **241**, 1483–6.

McMahon, B. (1993) Tackling stress at its roots. *Community Psychiatric Nursing Journal*, **13**(4), 30–1.

Mendlson, L. (1993a) Closing days (part 1). *Community Psychiatric Nursing Journal*, **13**(4), 23–9.

Mendlson, L. (1993b) Closing days (part 2). *Community Psychiatric Nursing Journal*, **13**(5), 22–7.

Meyer, E. (1962) Disturbed behaviour on medical and surgical wards, in *Science and Psychoanalysis*, Vol. 5, (ed. J. Masserman), Grune and Stratton, New York.

Meyer, E. and Mendelson, M. (1961) Psychiatric consultation with patients on a medical and surgical ward: patterns and processes. *Psychiatry*, **24**, 197–220.

Moos, R.H. and Insel, P.M. (1981) *Manual for the Work Environment Scale*, Consulting Psychologists Press, California.

Nichols, K.A., Springford, V. and Searle, J. (1981) An investigation of distress and discontent in various types of nursing. *Journal of Advanced Nursing*, **6**, 311–18.

Payne, R.L. (1979) Demands, supports, constraints and psychological health, in *Response to Stress: Occupational Aspects* (eds C.J. Mackay and T. Cox), International Publishing Company, London.

Payne, R. and Firth-Cozens, J. (1987) *Stress in Health Professionals*, John Wiley and Sons, Chichester.

Peat, L. and Watt, G. (1984) The passing of an era. *Community Psychiatric Nursing Journal*, **4**(2), 12–16.

Power, K.G. and Sharp, G.R. (1988) A comparison of sources of nursing stress and job satisfaction among mental handicap and hospice nursing staff. *Journal of Advanced Nursing*, **13**, 726–32.

Rees, D.W. and Smith, S.D. (1991) Work stress in occupational therapists assessed by the Occupational Stress Indicator. *British Journal of Occupational Therapy*, **54**(8), 289–94.

Rosenberg, M. (1965) *Society and the Adolescent Self-Image*, Princeton University Press, Princeton.

Rump, E.E. (1979) Size of psychiatric hospitals and nurses' job satisfaction. *Journal of Occupational Psychology*, **52**, 255–65.

Russell, A.T., Pasnau, R.O. and Traintor, Z.C. (1975) Emotional problems of residents in psychiatry. *American Journal of Psychiatry*, **132**(3), 263–7.

Rutter, M. (1981) Coping and development: some issues and some questions. *Journal of Child Psychology and Psychiatry*, **22**, 323–56.

Schafer, T. (1992) CPN stress and organisational change: a study. *Community Psychiatric Nursing Journal*, **12**(1), 16–24.

Seecombe, I. and Buchan, J. (1993) *Absent Nurses: The Costs and Consequences*, Institute of Manpower Studies, UK.

Skidmore, D. and Friend, W. (1985) Should CPNs be in the primary health care team? *Nursing Times*, Community Outlook, 310–12.

Sweeney, G.M., Nicholls, K.A. and Kline, P. (1991) Factors contributing to work-related stress in occupational therapists: results from a pilot study. *British Journal of Occupational Therapy*, **54**(8), 284–8.

Vreeland, R. and Ellis, G.L. (1969) Stresses on the nurse in an intensive-care unit. *Journal of the Americn Medical Association*, **208**, 332–4.

West, M., Jones, A. and Savage, Y. (1988) Stress in health visiting: a quantitative assessment. *Health Visitor*, **61**, 269–71.

White, E. (1990) *The Third Quinquennial National Community Psychiatric Nursing Survey*, Department of Nursing, University of Manchester.

CHAPTER 6

Findings from the Claybury study for ward based psychiatric nurses and comparisons with community psychiatric nurses

John Leary and Daniel Brown

INTRODUCTION

As mentioned in previous chapters the emphasis of the Claybury study was an examination of the stress levels experienced by community psychiatric nurses (CPNs) and ward based psychiatric nurses (WBPNs) in the course of carrying out their work. The study also provided the opportunity to examine the effectiveness of various procedures which nurses might utilize in attempting to cope with such occupational stress.

This chapter will concentrate on presenting the findings for the WBPNs in terms of the effect which occupational stress has on the degree of satisfaction which they experience within their work, the extent of occupational burnout which they experience along with their levels of general health and their utilization of coping strategies and the effectiveness of such strategies. Also included within this chapter are comparisons between the findings obtained for the CPNs (detailed more fully in Chapter 7) and those obtained for the ward based nurses. This chapter will therefore contain the following sections:

1. comparisons of personal demographic data for CPNs and WBPNs;
2. comparisons of professional demographic data for CPNs and WBPNs;

3. results obtained for WBPNs on stress related measures;
4. comparisons of results obtained for CPNs and WBPNs;
5. an examination of the characteristics of WBPNs who utilize coping strategies;
6. an examination of the effectiveness of the use of coping strategies for WBPNs;
7. predicting occupational burnout, job satisfaction and general health for WBPNs.

The WBPNs who participated in the study came from seven psychiatric hospitals and DGH units in the North East Thames Region. A total of 323 ward based psychiatric nurses were surveyed. This is a difficult time for hospital psychiatric nursing staff as hospitals are rapidly closing and jobs that once appeared to be 'jobs for life' are now under immediate threat. There were times when suspicion and reluctance to be involved in the study were encountered by the researcher. One ward manager succinctly explained that:

> The nursing staff have a lot going on at the moment. They are worried about job security and their places on the wards. They find many of the questions very personal and do not want to answer them. Also, however irrational, they feel that there may be an ulterior motive behind the questionnaires.

Overall, however, ward nurses were enthusiastic about the research and deeply concerned about the current changes occurring in NHS mental health services. Despite the length of the questionnaires, nurses were willing to use time out from busy schedules to answer a wide range of difficult questions. We are grateful to everyone who has participated and helped to generate a large sample from which we hope we have gleaned useful information. Our hope is that this information will serve a constructive purpose for all the psychiatric nurses who have taken part, for the wider community of UK psychiatric nurses and for patient care.

COMPARISON OF PERSONAL DEMOGRAPHIC DATA FOR WBPNs AND CPNs

In terms of the personal demographic data obtained from the participants of the Claybury Stress Study there proved to be a remarkable similarity between the CPN sample and the WBPN sample. The mean average age of WBPNs was 34.7 years with the youngest aged 18 years and the eldest 64 years (Table 6.1). The CPN sample obtained a slightly higher average age of 38.9 years but had a smaller range of ages (22–57 years) which would appear to reflect the career path

Table 6.1 Comparison of personal demographic data for WBPNs (n = 323) and CPNs (n = 250)

		WBPNs	*CPNs*
Age	Mean	34.7	38.9
	SD	9.7	7.9
Gender	Male	120 (37.2%)	95 (38%)
	Female	203 (62.8%)	155 (62%)
Marital status	Married/cohabiting	210 (65%)	185 (74%)
	Unmarried/separated	113 (35%)	65 (26%)
Dependants	Children at home	154 (47.7%)	136 (54.4%)
	No children at home	169 (52.3%)	114 (45.6%)

taken by CPNs who have usually gained initial psychiatric experience working within hospital settings before going on to work in the community. This is highlighted by the findings that only 3.6% of the CPN sample was aged 25 years or under compared to 19.2% of WBPNs. There is also an indication of the older, more experienced WBPNs transferring over to community based psychiatric work with only 26.3% of WBPNs aged 40 years or over compared to 36.4% of CPNs.

A virtually identical gender ratio was obtained between both nursing groups with the WBPNs comprising 203 (62.8%) females and 120 (37.2%) males compared to approximately 62% and 38% respectively within the CPN sample. Proportionally fewer of the WBPNs were married or cohabiting with a partner compared to CPNs (65% and 73% respectively) which reflects the younger age group of the ward based nurses. Of the subjects within the WBPN sample 154 (47.7%) had dependent children living at home compared to 54% of CPNs.

COMPARISON OF PROFESSIONAL DEMOGRAPHIC DATA FOR WBPNs AND CPNs

As can be seen from Table 6.2 there is a striking difference in the professional grading structure of both nursing groups with the hospital based nurses having only 34 of the participants, which represents 10.5% of their sample, positioned on Grade G or higher, while examination of the CPN grading structure shows that 82.2% of CPNs are ranked on or above a G Grade.

Ward based nurses had a mean average of 10.3 years of psychiatric work experience compared to 15.2 years for CPNs with 70% of CPNs

Table 6.2 Nursing grades of WBPNs and CPNs in percentages.

	Grade								
	A	B	C	D	E	F	G	H	I
WBPN	23.8	4.3	0.6	24.5	26.7	9.6	9.9	0.3	0.3
CPN	0	1.2	0.4	0.8	2.4	9.9	65.1	12.7	4.4

Table 6.3 Results obtained on stress related measures completed by WBPNs

	Mean	SD	Range
JOB SATISFACTION			
Total	62.6	11.7	20–92
Intrinsic	40.1	7.3	12–59
Extrinsic	16.5	4.6	6–44
OCCUPATIONAL BURNOUT			
Emotional exhaustion	20.4	12.0	0–50
Depersonalization	7.3	6.2	0–37
Personal accomplishment	32.3	8.5	5–48
SELF-ATTITUDE	16.9	4.6	10–31
GHQ	3.4	4.8	0–23

having over ten years experience compared to only 41% of WBPNs. Although both groups of nurses averaged approximately five years in their current post 47.2% of the CPN sample felt that they had good job security in their current position compared to only 28.8% of the hospital based psychiatric nurses.

RESULTS OBTAINED FOR WBPNs ON STRESS RELATED MEASURES

As indicated in previous chapters a number of measures were used in the Claybury study to examine the stressful effects of working in psychiatric nursing and also to look at the degree to which various coping strategies are utilized in attempting to alleviate such stress. The results obtained for measures which relate to the possible effects of stress are summarized in Table 6.3.

The Minnesota Job Satisfaction Scale (Koelbel *et al.*, 1991) was used to assess the levels of satisfaction experienced by nurses in the process of carrying out their jobs. The total job satisfaction score has a maximum range of 20–100 with higher scores representing greater levels of satisfaction. Ward based psychiatric nurses obtained a mean average total score of 62.6 which would place them in the mid-range of possible scores, indicating a somewhat neutral attitude towards their job with their posts being viewed as neither particularly satisfying or dissatisfying. This average score of total job satisfaction obtained by WBPNs does, however, disguise the distribution of scores obtained with only 35.9% of nurses scoring within the 'dissatisfied' range of scores.

The Minnesota Satisfaction Scale also allows examination of intrinsic and extrinsic job satisfaction. The intrinsic subscale, which has a range of 12–60, deals with factors such as the degree of responsibility nurses experience within their post, the degree of recognition they feel they receive and their perceived sense of achievement with regards to the work which they carry out. The extrinsic subscale, which has a range of 6–30, deals with factors such as salary, job image and job status. Ward based psychiatric nurses obtained an average intrinsic job satisfaction score of 40.1 which falls just inside the 'satisfied' half of the possible range of scores. However, 70% of the WBPN's scores fell within this half. The extrinsic subscale achieved an average score of 16.5 for WBPNs and represents over 60% of the sample falling within the 'dissatisfied' half of the possible range.

The results obtained from the Minnesota Satisfaction Scale would seem to suggest that the majority of ward based nurses experience to some degree feelings of satisfaction with the nature of the work which they carry out although there would appear to be a proportion who are actually highly dissatisfied. Additionally, however, many feel dissatisfied with extrinsic factors which do not relate to what they actually do but more to how they perceive themselves as being treated by their managers, employers and society in general.

The Maslach Burnout Inventory (Maslach and Jackson, 1986), which examines aspects of occupational burnout, contains three subscales covering the extent to which individuals feel emotionally exhausted by their work, how detached or depersonalized they become from the clients they work with and the degree of personal accomplishment with their work that they experience. The mean average score obtained for WBPNs in terms of emotional exhaustion was 20.4 which falls on the border between average and high burnout for mental health workers, with 44% of WBPNs assessed as experiencing high emotional burnout within their post. The depersonalization average score of 7.3 places WBPNs again on the border between average and high levels of depersonalization with 40.9% experiencing high levels of detached interaction with their patients. In terms of achieving a sense of personal accomplishment with their work, the mean WBPNs score of 32.3 indicates an average level of personal accomplishment which one would expect to find for mental health workers although

48.6% of the sample were assessed as experiencing low levels of occupational accomplishment.

Overall the results obtained from the Maslach Burnout Inventory for ward based psychiatric nurses would seem to indicate the need for some concern regarding the professional occupational situation which ward based nurses currently find themselves in and how they themselves perceive this situation. While the mean average scores for both emotional exhaustion and depersonalization fell in the average to high range, over 40% of the nursing sample were actually scoring in the high burnout range on both subscales. The extent of high burnout regarding personal accomplishment approached 50% of the ward based participants (Table 6.4).

Table 6.4 Percentage of WBPNs experiencing occupational burnout

	Occupational burnout		
	High	*Average*	*Low*
Emotional exhaustion	44.0	21.3	34.7
Personal accomplishment	48.6	20.4	31.0
Depersonalization	40.9	21.9	37.2

The self-attitude or self-esteem of WBPNs was assessed by means of the Rosenberg Self-Attitude Scale (Rosenberg, 1965). This scale has a maximum range of scores of 10–40. Scores below 17 are generally thought to reflect positive views of oneself whereas scores above 21 are considered to be somewhat negative. The mean average score obtained by WBPNs was 16.9 which would place it on the border between average and positive self-attitude. The results obtained indicated that over half of the WBPNs who participated in the study had positive views of themselves whereas just over 20% viewed themselves negatively.

The general health of WBPNs was assessed using the General Health Questionnaire (Goldberg and Williams, 1988) which has a maximum possible range of scores of 0–28 with a recommended threshold score of five or above as an indication of 'psychiatric caseness'. The mean average score obtained by WBPNs was 3.4; however, 27.9% of these nurses obtained scores above the threshold. This would appear to be a matter of some concern with the indication being that over one quarter of the nursing staff caring for psychiatric patients in hospital settings are themselves fulfilling criteria indicating psychiatric caseness.

COMPARISON OF RESULTS OBTAINED FOR
CPNs AND WBPNs

Stress related measures

Apart from the CPN Stress Questionnaire (Brown *et al.*, 1994), which only the CPN group completed, all other measures were completed by both groups of nurses which therefore provided the opportunity for comparisons to be made between the CPNs and the WBPNs. The comparisons carried out on the stress related measures are summarized in Table 6.5.

Table 6.5 Comparison of mean scores for WBPNs and CPNs

	WBPNs	CPNs	Significance*
GHQ	3.4	4.8	p<.05
OCCUPATIONAL BURNOUT			
Emotional exhaustion	20.4	21.5	NS
Depersonalization	7.3	5.4	p<.0001
Personal accomplishment	32.3	34.4	p<.005
JOB SATISFACTION			
Total	62.6	66.1	p<.0005
Intrinsic	40.1	44.1	p<.0001
Extrinsic	16.5	16.4	NS
SELF-ATTITUDE	16.9	16.6	NS

*Mann-Whitney test

The results obtained from the General Health Questionnaire indicated that the CPNs obtained significantly higher GHQ scores than did WBPNs and indeed 41% of the total CPN sample passed the threshold for psychiatric caseness on this measure compared to almost 28% of the hospital based nurses. The findings for both nursing groups are worryingly high and indicate the importance of attempting to evaluate what it is within each profession that contributes to such large proportions of both nursing groups achieving psychiatric caseness criteria.

At first glance it may seem intuitively reasonable to assume that the length of time which individuals spent working in such a demanding profession as nursing may contribute in determining their level of well-being, with nurses of longer durations faring less well than those of shorter durations. CPNs obtain significantly higher scores on the GHQ than WBPNs and as indicated earlier, the majority of CPNs arrive at their position after having gained psychiatric experience on hospital psychiatric wards and have therefore on average accumulated longer durations of nursing experience than WBPNs. However, a multiple regression analysis (described in more detail later) indicated that duration of experience was not a significant factor in predicting GHQ outcome for WBPNs. The explanation for such high scores on the GHQ would appear to lie within components of the work itself, the degree of support obtained and individuals' self-perception rather than length of experience.

Significant differences between CPNs and WBPNs were also detected in two of the subscales on the Maslach Burnout Inventory. There was a much higher rate of feelings of depersonalization or detachment from their patients for hospital based psychiatric nurses, with 41% of them assessed as experiencing high depersonalization burnout as opposed to the significantly lower proportion of 24% of CPNs. In terms of personal accomplishment WBPNs again obtained a significantly higher burnout rate with 31% of them reporting low feelings of personal accomplishment as opposed to 20% of the CPNs. Although there was no significant difference obtained between the two groups on the emotional exhaustion subscale, large proportions of both groups reported significant levels of burnout with 48% of CPNs and 44% of WBPNs experiencing high levels of emotional exhaustion.

The results obtained from this measure of occupational burnout present a picture of the two groups of nurses feeling emotionally exhausted by the current demands of their profession. At present, however, the ward based nurses are reporting higher levels of burnout than CPNs in as much as they experience significantly less personal accomplishment and significantly higher feelings of depersonalization from their own patient group.

In terms of feelings of satisfaction with their current work, CPNs displayed a significantly higher degree of job satisfaction. This, however, was largely explained by their greater sense of satisfaction with factors intrinsic to their profession such as their perceived sense of achievement, the recognition they receive for their efforts and the degree of responsibility they feel they hold. No significant difference was obtained between the two nursing groups with regards to factors extrinsic to the profession such as salary and the perceived status of the job.

Additionally there was no significant difference detected in the self-attitude of nurses in both nursing groups. Ward based psychiatric nurses obtained an average score of 16.9 compared to 16.6 for CPNs. These scores would indicate that nurses in both professions, on average, have a balanced view of themselves, recognizing both their good and bad points and tending to be somewhat positive in terms of competence and self-value. However, although the group averages of self-attitude tend to be quite encouraging, 14.6% of WBPNs and

18% of CPNs still tended to view themselves negatively and felt that others do not hold much respect for them.

Coping strategy measures

Information obtained from a demographic questionnaire used in the study indicated a number of methods utilized by nurses in their attempts to reduce occupational stress. Of the 323 ward based nurses who participated in the study, 287 (88.9%) felt that they could discuss work related problems with their work colleagues as a means of alleviating work related stress. There was no significant difference in the usage of this strategy between the two different nursing groups, with 92.8% of CPNs also feeling that they could discuss their work related problems with colleagues.

There was, however, a significant difference in the extent that CPNs and WBPNs felt that they were supported by their line managers. A combined total of 63 (19.6%) WBPNs considered their line manager to be unsupportive with 5% feeling them to be very unsupportive. This compares with 57 (22.8%) of CPNs reporting unsupportive managers with 4.8% reporting them to be very unsupportive (Table 6.6).

The stressful nature of the work carried out by both nursing professions produced no significant difference in the amount of time taken off work over the past 12 months, although 18.6% of WBPNs had taken ten or more days sick leave over the past year compared to 14.8% of CPNs. In terms of alcohol consumption as a means of reducing the stressful pressures of work, 46 (14.2%) hospital based psychiatric nurses reported never drinking alcohol while 13 (4.0%) reported drinking over 21 units per week. No significant difference was detected between consumption levels between WBPNs and CPNs. In terms of cigarette consumption, however, a highly significant difference between the two nursing groups was obtained with ward based nurses more likely to smoke and more likely to smoke heavily.

A coping skills questionnaire (Cooper *et al.*, 1988) was used to estimate the extent that both nursing groups utilized various coping strategies which had been identified as beneficial in attempting to reduce occupation related stress. Additionally, this also allowed a comparison to be made between both nursing groups in their use of such strategies.

The Coping Skills Questionnaire covers six distinct subscales each identified as a possible source of coping with stress. These are defined as:

1. **Social support**. The degree of support either direct or indirect which is received from others.

Table 6.6 Methods of reducing stress reported in the demographic questionnaire for WBPNs and CPNs

	WBPNs	*CPNs*	*Significance**
CIGARETTES			
None	199 (61.6%)	183 (73.2%)	
1–20	95 (29.4%)	53 (21.2%)	p<.005
Over 20	29 (9.0%)	14 (5.6%)	
ALCOHOL			
None	46 (14.2%)	29 (11.6%)	
Under 21 units weekly	264 (81.8%)	215 (86.0%)	NS
Over 21 units weekly	13 (4%)	6 (2.4%)	
DISCUSS PROBLEMS WITH WORK COLLEAGUES	287 (88.9%)	232 (92.8%)	NS**
SUPPORTIVE MANAGER			
Very supportive	125 (38.7%)	69 (27.6%)	
Supportive	135 (41.8%)	124 (49.6%)	p<.05
Unsupportive	47 (14.6%)	45 (18%)	
Very unsupportive	16 (5.0%)	12 (4.8%)	
ABSENCE FROM WORK DURING PAST YEAR			
None	91 (28.2%)	67 (26.8%)	
1–10 days	172 (53.2%)	146 (58.4%)	NS
11–20 days	32 (10.0%)	21 (8.4%)	
Over 20 days	28 (8.6%)	16 (6.4%)	

*Mann-Whitney test
**Chi square test

2. **Task strategies**. The degree to which individuals reorganize their work, either on an immediate micro level or on a wider macro level.
3. **Logic**. The degree of objectivity achieved and the adoption of an unemotional and rational approach to one's work.
4. **Home and work relationships**. The degree to which an individual's personal home life helps to alleviate stress generated at work.
5. **Time**. The efficient management of an individual's time in relation to the work demands placed on them.
6. **Involvement**. The degree to which individuals commit themselves to the work situation, thereby promoting the possibility of viewing the situation as it really is or 'coming to terms with reality'.

The results of the Coping Skills Questionnaire for WBPNs and CPNs showed a remarkable similarity between both groups in terms of the degree to which they both utilize these distinct coping strategies (Table 6.7). Two of the measures, 'task strategies' and 'logic' achieved

Table 6.7 Comparison of Coping Skills Questionnaire results for WBPNs and CPNs

	CPN		WBPN		
	Mean	*SD*	*Mean*	*SD*	*Significance**
Social support	18.0	3.1	17.7	3.5	NS
Task strategies	26.7	3.9	27.9	4.9	p<.005
Logic	12.1	2.0	12.7	2.4	p<.005
Home & work relationships	17.9	3.7	17.7	3.6	NS
Time	15.3	2.3	15.0	2.6	NS
Involvement	24.7	3.2	25.2	3.9	NS

*Mann-Whitney test

a statistically significant difference; however, their mean average scores were very similar as indeed were their mode average scores (27 for CPNs and 28 for WBPNs with regards to 'task strategies' and 12 for both groups for 'logic'). The statistical significance may be explained by the wider range of scores achieved by the hospital based nurses which would tend to make the usefulness of such a finding questionable. All of the remaining coping strategy procedures demonstrated virtually identical mean average scores for both nursing groups.

In an attempt to evaluate whether any of the six coping strategy subscales were utilized more productively by either of the two nursing groups, further analysis was carried out with the aim of assessing whether the use of particular coping strategies had different consequences for WBPNs and CPNs. Within the study being reported such differences in consequences refer to the outcome on measures such as the General Health Questionnaire and the Maslach Burnout Inventory for each of the nursing groups.

Examination of interaction results obtained from analysis of variance indicated that there were no significant differences between both nursing groups with regards to their use of all six coping strategies and the consequential outcome on the GHQ, their experience of depersonalization and their sense of personal accomplishment. Significant differences were obtained, however, with regards to the level of emotional exhaustion each group experienced and the degree to which they utilized the coping strategies of 'time management' and 'task strategies'. As Figure 6.1 shows, the practice of time management for hospital based psychiatric nurses had little effect on the level of emotional exhaustion they reported. For CPNs, however, there is a clear and significant relationship between a lower use of time management as a coping strategy to stress and an increase in the level of emotional exhaustion experienced. Such findings may reflect the

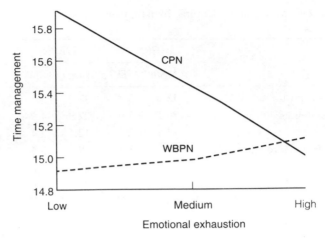

Figure 6.1 Interaction between the coping strategy of time management and emotional exhaustion for WBPNs and CPNs.

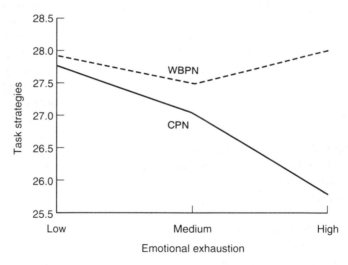

Figure 6.2 Interaction between the use of task stratregies as a means of coping and emotional exhaustion for WBPNs and CPNs.

extent to which CPNs work autonomously and as such highlight the importance of the efficient use of their time as without such efficiency work related stress may occur and with it greater feelings of emotional exhaustion. Ward based nurses, on the other hand, are more closely integrated within a team and as such time management practices are more likely to be designed at a team level as opposed to the level of individual workers. Without the same degree of control over their time as CPNs have, hospital nurses are less likely to feel that time is an issue of stress. Consequently it would appear that for WBPNs time management and emotional exhaustion do not display a similar relationship to that found for CPNs.

A similar picture was also obtained with regards to the use of 'task strategies' as a means of coping with stress. Figure 6.2 once again shows the emotional exhaustion of CPNs increasing in relation to a decrease in the utilization of task strategies as a method of coping with stress. For the WBPNs, however, the use of task strategies did not appear to influence the degree of emotional exhaustion experienced. This finding may again reflect the degree to which CPNs are required to work efficiently on their own largely without the benefit of team work practices and task structures. If they fail to generate their own task strategies for the work that they carry out there would appear to be a greater likelihood of increased feelings of emotional exhaustion.

EXAMINATION OF THE CHARACTERISTICS OF WBPNs WHO UTILIZE COPING STRATEGIES

Additional analysis of the data obtained from WBPNs was carried out to examine whether there were detectable differences in the personal and professional characteristics of hospital based nurses who made high or low use of the various coping strategies.

Social support

A number of significant differences were found between WBPNs who utilized social support as a means of coping with occupationally related stress and those who did not (Table 6.8). Unsurprisingly a significantly larger number of WBPNs who did not utilize social support as a means of coping with stress were found to be unmarried. Social support is not, however, exclusively a reflection of marital status, it relates also the extent which supportive relationships in general exist and such relationships can also include professional relationships. Indeed, WBPNs with low social support were significantly more likely to feel that their manager was unsupportive and a significantly higher proportion of WBPNs also felt that they were unable to discuss problems with their work colleagues.

Low social support scorers were also more likely to feel unhappy with their life and they were also more likely to view themselves critically and be negative in their self-attitudes. Low use of this coping strategy was also significantly related to experiencing higher levels of emotional exhaustion and lower levels of personal accomplishment

Table 6.8 Differences between high and low users of social support as a means of coping for WBPNs

	Social support		Significance*
	High	Low	
UNMARRIED (n)	28	73	p<.05**
UNSUPPORTIVE MANAGER	1.7	2.0	p<.01
UNABLE TO DISCUSS PROBLEMS WITH COLLEAGUES	9(30%)	21 (70%)	p<.05
HAPPINESS WITH LIFE	3.9	3.5	p<.001
EMOTIONAL EXHAUSTION	18.2	21.8	p<.05
PERSONAL ACCOMPLISHMENT	33.3	30.5	p<.05
JOB SATISFACTION			
Total	64.5	60.4	p<.05
Intrinsic	41.6	38.5	p<.05
SELF-ATTITUDE	16.0	17.5	p<.005

*Mann-Whitney test
**Chi square test

indicating a greater likelihood of occupational burnout. Low scorers of social support were also significantly more likely to report lower levels of satisfaction with their work.

Task strategies

The use of task strategies as a means of coping with occupational stress reflects the degree to which WBPNs organize their work patterns both on an immediate, personal level and on a more indirect, global level. Significantly hospital based nurses who made greater use of this strategy were more likely to have obtained an RMN qualification (Table 6.9) indicating perhaps the importance of professional training in providing individuals with the knowledge of organizational patterns and structures which promote efficient methods of work. Nurses who utilized this coping strategy were also more likely to feel happier with their lives than those who did not. Interestingly, they were also more likely to drink significantly less alcohol, smoke significantly fewer cigarettes and regard themselves as fitter than WBPNs who did not utilize task strategies within their work.

Significant differences were also detected in the degree of occupational burnout experienced by high and low users of this strategy. Those who utilized the strategy were assessed as experiencing low levels of burnout in that they experienced greater feelings of personal accomplishment regarding their work.

Table 6.9 Differences between high and low users of task strategies as a means of coping for WBPNs

| | Task strategies | | |
	High	Low	Significance*
RMN	55.4%	44.6%	p<.05**
Fitness	2.0	2.3	p<.001
Alcohol	3.1	2.9	p<.05
Cigarettes	1.6	1.9	p<.05
Happiness with life	3.8	3.5	p<.01
Personal accomplishment	34.0	30.1	p<.0005

*Mann-Whitney test
**Chi square test

Table 6.10 Differences between high and low users of logic as a means of coping for WBPNs

| | Logic | | |
	High	Low	Significance
RMN	59.7%	40.3%	p<.05**
Unable to discuss problems with work colleagues	74.1%	25.9%	p<.05*

*Mann-Whitney test
**Chi square test

Logic

WBPNs who made use of a logical approach to their work as a means of reducing stress differed significantly on only two variables compared to those who did not utilize logic as a means of coping. As we would perhaps expect, nurses with a completed RMN training were more likely to take a logical approach to their work than nurses without an RMN in as much as they were more likely to adopt an unemotional and rational approach to the task at hand (Table 6.10).

Somewhat surprisingly, however, WBPNs who made use of logic in their work were significantly less likely to discuss problems with their work colleagues. The reasoning for this may possibly be that in the process of adopting a logical approach to work tasks there is to some extent a suppression of one's own feelings while attempting to be objective. In such a way individuals who make use of a logical approach may feel that difficulties experienced in the course of their work are difficulties inherent to the task at hand and as such do not reflect upon themselves. They may consequently feel that they should get on with the job at hand as opposed to discussing it with others. It is of interest that such a 'logic' approach to work would appear to differ from the use of 'social support' as a means of coping with stress and indeed the correlational relationship between the two coping strategies was only 0.22 and was the lowest found between any of the coping strategies investigated.

Home and work relationship

The extent to which individuals feel content in their personal life can also influence the degree to which they cope with their work situation. As such the relationship between home life and work can be regarded as a coping strategy in its own right. WBPNs who achieved high scores on this scale would consider themselves as living a rich and varied home life whereas low scorers would tend to feel that their personal home life was presently unsatisfactory. As would be expected there was a significant difference between high and low scoring WBPNs in terms of how happy they felt about their present life with high scorers on the home and work relationship scale feeling significantly happier (Table 6.11). Hospital based nurses with a satisfactory personal life were also significantly more likely to have a positive self-image and to be less critical of themselves. High scorers were also more likely to report greater feelings of personal accomplishment concerning their work compared to low scoring WBPNs.

Table 6.11 Differences between high and low scorers on home and work relationship as a means of coping for WBPNs

	Home and work relationship		
	High	Low	Significance*
Happiness with life	3.8	3.6	p<.05
Self-attitude	15.9	17.6	p<.01
Fitness	2.2	2.3	p<.01
Personal accomplishment	33.1	30.4	p<.05
Job satisfaction (extrinsic)	15.9	17.5	p<.005

*Mann-Whitney test

Time management

The effective management of one's time is perhaps one of the most obvious methods of increasing one's own professional efficiency, thereby reducing the potential pressure and stress of the job. However, regardless of its intuitive effectiveness as a coping strategy it would appear that it is not universally practised and significant differences appear to exist between WBPNs who utilize time management to alleviate stress within their work and those who do not (Table 6.12). The age of WBPNs was found to differ significantly between high and low users of time management with high users tending to be older and having more psychiatric work experience than low users. High users were also more likely to have a greater sense of personal accomplishment than low users and although the high users were on average older they also considered themselves to be fitter than low users.

Table 6.12 Differences between high and low use of time management as a means of coping for WBPNs

| | *Time management* | | |
	High	*Low*	*Significance**
Age	35.6	32.9	p<.01
Duration of experience	11.0	9.2	p<.05
Fitness	2.1	2.3	p<.005
Cigarettes	1.6	2.0	p<.005
Personal accomplishment	32.8	29.8	p<.05

*Mann-Whitney test

Involvement

The last of the coping strategies which was investigated was that of becoming involved or immersing oneself in the job in hand (Table 6.13). WBPNs who utilized this strategy by having a high commitment to the job differed from those who did not by tending, once again, to

Table 6.13 Differences between high and low involvement with work as a means of coping for WBPNs

| | *Involvement* | | |
	High	*Low*	*Significance**
Age	36.2	33.7	p<.05
Fitness	1.9	2.4	p<.0001
Alcohol	3.1	2.9	p<.05
Cigarettes	1.6	1.9	p<.05
GHQ	2.9	4.2	p<.05
Personal accomplishment	33.4	30.5	p<.05

*Mann-Whitney test

be older and reporting higher levels of personal accomplishment. Higher involvement in the job also related to significantly lower and better scores on the GHQ along with higher levels of fitness than those who were less involved in their work. Such involvement or submergence into one's work was also related to significantly lower intake levels of both alcohol and tobacco.

THE EFFECTIVENESS OF THE USE OF COPING STRATEGIES FOR WBPNs

Although the Coping Skills Questionnaire has proved useful in identifying different coping strategy procedures, at present one of its limitations would appear to be that the normative studies carried out on it have used business managers as their sample and it is questionable as to whether such normative data could usefully be applied to mental health workers. As such, it is difficult to determine exactly what the scores obtained on the different subscales actually signify; that is, we currently do not know what a mental health nurse would on average be expected to score on each scale given the uniqueness of their profession and the difficulties inherent in it.

Comparisons have already been reported between high and low users of such coping strategies for WBPNs as well as comparisons between CPNs and WBPNs. These comparisons, however, elucidate only whether one group uses the various coping strategies more than another group and what factors appear to relate to such use. They do not explain whether the strategies being used have any beneficial effect on actually reducing the degree of stress experienced at work.

Consequently the data for WBPNs was further examined to determine whether the various coping strategies had an influence on the well-being of hospital based nurses. A comparison was made between WBPNs who made high or low use of the various coping strategies to determine whether there was a difference between their scores on the outcome measures such as the General Health Questionnaire and the Maslach Burnout Inventory (Table 6.14).

The results obtained indicated that five of the coping strategies were significantly related to hospital nurses sensing higher levels of personal accomplishment concerning their work. Only the use of 'logic' failed to improve WBPNs' feelings of competence and achievement.

The most successful coping strategy in terms of reducing the degree of emotional exhaustion was the use of 'social support'. Nurses who made low use of social support, whether in their private or professional life, were significantly more likely to suffer from high levels of emotional exhaustion.

Table 6.14 Significant differences obtained on the General Health Questionnaire, emotional exhaustion, depersonalization and personal accomplishment scales by WBPNs who make high or low use of coping strategies

	GHQ	EE	DP	PA
SOCIAL SUPPORT				
High		18.2		33.3
Low		21.8*		30.5*
TASK STRATEGIES				
High				34.0
Low				30.1**
LOGIC				
High				
Low				
HOME AND WORK RELATIONSHIP				
High				33.1
Low				30.4*
TIME MANAGEMENT				
High				32.8
Low				29.8*
INVOLVEMENT				
High	2.9			33.4
Low	4.2*			30.5*

* p < .05
** p < .0005
Mann-Whitney test

Interestingly, the use of 'involvement' was found to be significantly related to lower GHQ scores. It may, however, be somewhat inaccurate to interpret this result as signifying that higher involvement leads to an improvement in one's general health rating. Although higher involvement may well contribute to good general health (and vice versa) it is likely that there are other factors operating in people's lives which may influence not only the likelihood of their being very involved in their work but also their general state of health. Perhaps what this finding does signify is that when nurses find themselves in a position where they are able to submerge themselves into their work they are generally in a good state of health.

None of the various coping strategies succeeded in producing significant differences in the degree of depersonalization which WBPNs experienced. This is a highly disappointing finding, particularly when we consider that over 40% of WBPNs were reported to be experiencing high levels of depersonalization burnout.

PREDICTING OCCUPATIONAL BURNOUT, JOB
SATISFACTION AND GENERAL HEALTH FOR WBPNs

In an attempt to examine the relationship between the coping strategies outlined and the outcome measures used in the study, the data for ward based psychiatric nurses were subjected to correlational analysis (Table 6.15). The results obtained indicated an array of significant but extremely low correlations between the variables under investigation. The use of 'logic' and 'time management' by WBPNs as strategies for coping with stress were found not to correlate significantly with any of the outcome measures used, indicating perhaps the degree to which the work of the hospital based nurse is strongly located within that of a team. The overall picture obtained would appear to be one of a complex combination of coping strategies required to alleviate the stress of work. Individual strategies in isolation are not effective in producing change but seem to need to be used in combination with other strategies and indeed, further as yet unidentified coping stratgies may be required in order to decrease the degree of depersonalization and increase the sense of job satisfaction, neither of which correlated with any of the coping strategies indicated.

The analysis of the data obtained from WBPNs has been useful in attempting to identify significant characteristic differences between subjects who appear to be suffering from the effects of occupational stress and those who appear to be coping. As such these findings attempt to develop our understanding of the links between work related stress and methods which appear to be particularly useful in reducing such stress.

It would, however, be additonally beneficial to gain insight into factors which appear to directly contribute towards the formation of stress in the first place. The old adage 'prevention is better than cure' is particularly relevant here in that there would be much sense in attempting to predict and anticipate the elements which contribute to the build-up of stress and thereby perhaps be in a position to prevent such stress occurring rather than attempting to reduce it once it has actually occurred.

The data obtained from WBPNs was therefore submitted to a stepwise multiple regression analysis to determine which factors act as the best predictors for the level of general health hospital nurses experience, their levels of occupational burnout and the degree of job satisfaction they experience.

Predictors of high GHQ scores

The stepwise multiple regression analysis indicated that six variables were the best predictors of GHQ scores for WBPNs.The overall R^2 of the equation was equal to 35.5%.The six predicting variables were:

Table 6.15 Significant correlations between outcome and coping strategy measures completed by WBPNs

	1	2	3	4	5	6	7	8	9	10	11	12	13	14
1. Grade														
2. GHQ														
3. Self-attitude		0.26												
4. Emotional exhaustion	0.12	0.46	0.22											
5. Depersonalization	0.12	0.32	0.19	0.6										
6. Personal accomplishment	0.14	−0.11	−0.27											
7. Job satisfaction total		−0.32	−0.23	−0.47	−0.32	0.15								
8. Job satisfaction intrinsic		−0.29	−0.28	−0.4	−0.26	0.19	0.91							
9. Job satisfaction extrinsic		−0.29	−0.14	−0.44	−0.3		0.86	0.62						
10. Social support		−0.13	−0.22	−0.12		0.15		0.14						
11. Task strategies	0.16		−0.14			0.21				0.48				
12. Logic									0.18	0.22	0.4			
13. Home/work relationships			−0.19			0.14				0.45	0.36	0.3		
14. Time management										0.33	0.48	0.33	0.27	
15. Involvement		−0.2	−0.16			0.15		0.14		0.47	0.59	0.33	0.4	0.42
	1	2	3	4	5	6	7	8	9	10	11	12	13	14

1. happiness with present life;
2. emotional exhaustion level;
3. fitness level;
4. intrinsic job satisfaction;
5. self-attitude;
6. number of patients.

Three of the predicting variables related directly to the work which individuals were involved in. The first of these predicting variables was the level of emotional exhaustion individuals experienced with their work, with high exhaustion predicting high GHQ scores. Low levels of satisfaction with factors intrinsic to their job further predicted a poor outcome on the GHQ questionnaire for WBPNs. Such intrinsic factors include the perceived degree of responsibility held by nurses and the levels of achievement attained with low levels of responsibility and a low sense of achievement predicting a high GHQ score. Additionally higher numbers of patients under the care of nurses also predicted poor GHQ outcome. Interestingly the three remaining predictors of GHQ scores for WBPNs relate to issues of their self-perception with particular focus on how happy they feel about their present life, how fit they consider themselves to be and whether they had a positive or negative view of themselves.

Predictors of high emotional exhaustion

Six variables were also found to be the best combination of predictors from the range of variables investigated within the study. The overall R^2 for this regression equation was equal to 29%. The six variables were:

1. total job satisfaction;
2. RMN;
3. self-attitude;
4. post-training qualifications;
5. intrinsic job satisfaction;
6. fitness level.

The strongest predictor of emotional exhaustion found for WBPNs was their overall satisfaction with their work with low levels of satisfaction relating to high levels of emotional burnout. The level of nursing qualification held was also found to be predictive in a particularly intriguing manner. Unqualified nurses were less likely than qualified nurses to be emotionally exhausted which may possibly be accounted for by higher levels of responsibility and longer periods of time in the job for the qualified staff. Interestingly, however, nurses who, once qualified, undertook additional training were also less likely to be emotionally exhausted than those who did not complete further training. This would seem to suggest that in predicting high levels of emotional exhaustion in WBPNs, particularly in qualified WBPNs, the extent to which they have developed their skills through further training should be taken into account. Once again nurses' perception of their own level of fitness was also found to be predictive of the degree of emotional exhaustion they report.

Predictors of high depersonalization and low personal accomplishment

Neither depersonalization or personal accomplishment was found to be highly predictive from the variables examined within this study with the overall R^2 for these equations being equal to 18% and 16% respectively. The strongest predictor of feelings of depersonalization which WBPNs had towards their work was the degree of overall satisfaction they experienced concerning their job with low levels of satisfaction leading to high feelings of depersonalization. An individual's sense of self-value was also a contributing factor with feelings of low self-value predicting a depersonalized approach to one's work. Self-value was also the strongest predictor for personal accomplishment, WBPNs with a sense of self-value achieving the greater sense of personal accomplishment. The nurses who feel personally accomplished would also tend to be qualified and experience satisfaction with factors intrinsic to their work.

Interestingly, however, individuals with a sense of personal accomplishment had a greater chance of being predicted not only by their use of the coping procedure of developing and utilizing task strategies within their work but also by their lack of the use of 'logic' or objectivity within their work as a coping strategy. This would seem to suggest that a rational and unemotional approach to one's work may help to reduce work related stress but does not necessarily lead to a greater sense of personal accomplishment.

Predictors of high job satisfaction

As one might expect there was a remarkable similarity across the variables which predicted total job satisfation, intrinsic job satisfaction and extrinsic job satisfaction. These obtained R^2 values equal to 37%, 27% and 34% respectively. The variables within the study which were found to be most predictive of total job satisfaction were:

1. supportive line manager;
2. emotional exhaustion level;
3. happiness with current life;

4. personal accomplishment level;
5. age;
6. job security.

The factor which was most predictive for all of the subscales of job satisfaction was the level of support nurses received from their managers. The more supportive mangers were, the greater the levels of satisfaction experienced by WBPNs. Low levels of emotional exhaustion were also found to be predictive of job satisfaction as was a sense of personal accomplishment with one's work and a sense of general happiness with one's life at present. The age of nurses was also found to be predictive with older nurses who felt that they had good job security within their current post being more satisfied with their post than those who felt little security within their post.

IMPLICATIONS OF FINDINGS FOR WARD BASED PSYCHIATRIC NURSES

The results obtained from the Claybury Stress Study for ward based psychiatric nurses would appear to reflect the difficult and unsettled times which the profession is currently experiencing, in particular with regard to the closure of psychiatric hospitals and the emergence of community based psychiatric care. The results indicate an air of discontent among WBPNs concerning this period of transition of care for hospital to community while there seem to be additional feelings of unease concerning the changes occurring within the NHS itself, particularly with the development of internal market forces through the introduction of the principles of the purchaser and the provider. The effect on WBPNs appears to be one of uncertainty regarding the future and disillusionment with the present.

The uncertainty of the future is perhaps highlighted by feelings of insecurity within their current posts with over 71% of WBPNs reporting that they felt that they did not have good job security, a much higher figure than that obtained from their community based counterparts. It is difficult to imagine individual nurses not being affected by such feelings of insecurity and the astonishingly high proportion who report such feelings would seem to underline a serious issue which needs to be addressed by health service managers.

Given the high levels of insecurity within their jobs, it is perhaps testimony to the dedication of nurses that the majority retain a sense of satisfaction with their work. From the results obtained, however, there appears to be a sizeable proportion who are highly dissatisfied with their work situation. Additionally although the majority of WBPNs gain satisfaction from their work their level of satisfaction is significantly less than that reported by community based nurses, particularly with regard to factors intrinsic to their work such as the recognition received for the work that they carry out and the degree of responsibility they hold. Interestingly, both groups of nurses were dissatisfied with extrinsic factors of the job such as salary and status, including issues such as the degree of respect received, sources of which could be the general public, service users and the health service authority themselves. It could perhaps be argued that the perceived lack of job security previously mentioned could contribute to the low extrinsic job satisfaction experienced by WBPNs.

The higher levels of job satisfaction experienced by CPNs compared to WBPNs are also reflected in the lower rates of occupational burnout experienced by CPNs compared to WBPNs. The hospital based nurses experienced a significantly lower level of personal accomplishment than the community based nurses and indeed almost half the WBPN sample reported experiencing low levels of personal accomplishment within their job. Hospital nurses also experienced a significantly greater level of depersonalization within their work while two out of every five WBPNs reported feeling highly emotionally exhausted by their work.

With such levels of occupational burnout it would perhaps be expected for the general health of WBPNs to be affected in some manner and indeed over one quarter of the WBPNs who participated in the study obtained scores on the GHQ which would place them above the recommended threshold of 'psychiatric caseness'.

From the results obtained it would therefore appear that there is a sizeable proportion of WBPNs who lack satisfaction within their work, are experiencing higher levels of occupational burnout than that found among their community based counter parts and are obtaining worryingly high results from the General Health Questionnaire which is indicating that they themselves are fulfilling criteria of 'psychiatric caseness' which would perhaps be more expected from the individuals they nurse and not from the nurses themselves.

The study attempted to examine factors which might be thought of as contributing towards such worryingly high GHQ scores, the identification of such factors being useful in attempting to predict or anticipate poor general health results. The findings indicate a number of work related factors which could be helpful in predicting poor general health outcome in WBPNs; these included experiencing high levels of emotional exhaustion, experiencing a lack of satisfaction with one's work and having large numbers of patients under one's care. Interestingly, attempts to identify factors which are useful in predicting occupational burnout in terms of emotional exhaustion revealed similar findings with low satisfaction with one's work contributing to high emotional exhaustion. Additional findings predicting emotional exhaustion, however, include a lack of further training once nurses had qualified, with qualified nurses who had not obtained further training achieving higher levels of emotional burnout than those who did obtain postqualification training.

Job satisfaction had been found to be useful in predicting levels of both general health and emotional exhaustion in WBPNs and could therefore be considered a useful yardstick of an individual's well-being. Consequently factors which were found to be most predictive of job satisfaction could, in a sense, contribute not only to job satisfaction but indirectly to the more general issues of WBPN's general well-being. Examination of the factors which contribute towards a good sense of job satisfaction indicated that the most predictive of these were a good sense of personal accomplishment with one's work, low levels of emotional exhaustion and a perception of one's line management as being supportive.

Attempting to predict any aspect of the future needs, of course, to take into account a complex arrangement of different factors which influence each other. At times, attempts to prevent or minimize predicted difficulties may be hampered by lack of choice or lack of influence by both nurses and their managers. However, some things may be more within reach than others. An example of this has been found to be the importance of receiving support from one's line management in increasing job satisfaction with the possible knock-on effect on levels of burnout and general health. Even if management do not have the power to significantly change the circumstances under which nurses work, they do have the opportunities to demonstrate support and understanding of the tremendous difficulties under which WBPNs often operate. The importance of supportive management is highlighted by findings that CPNs obtained significantly poorer general health results while considering that they also had significantly less supportive management.

Of the six coping strategies examined within the study, the only one which failed to contribute towards alleviating the differences of work proved to be the use of 'logic'. This would seem to suggest that the adoption of a purely objective and unemotional approach to one's work was unhelpful in attempting to significantly reduce work related stress. Indeed, higher 'involvement' with one's work, which was one of the other coping strategies investigated, proved to be more successful in alleviating occupational burnout and contributing towards improved general health. 'Involvement', or the degree to which individuals commit themselves to their work situation, was the only coping strategy which proved to be significantly related to general health with individuals who became highly involved in their work obtaining significantly better General Health Questionnaire scores. The coping strategy of 'social support' proved to be significant with regard to having an effect on emotional exhaustion and personal accomplishment, both of which are considered to be aspects of occupational burnout. WBPNs who received high levels of 'social support' were found to have significantly lower levels of emotional exhaustion compared to nurses who did not. They were also achieving a significantly higher score of personal accomplishment with their work. Indeed, personal accomplishment proved to be the most affected by a range of coping strategies including 'task strategies', 'time management' and 'home and work relationships' in addition to 'social support' and 'involvement'.

SUMMARY

The Claybury study of stress and coping strategies practised by psychiatric nurses indicated a number of interesting findings and comparisons between hospital based and community based nurses. Large proportions of both groups of nurses appear to experience high levels of emotional exhaustion due to the demands of their work. Additionally, ward based psychiatric nurses appear at present to experience greater feelings of depersonalization or detachment from their patients and less of a sense of personal accomplishment with their work compared to their community based counterparts. In the light of these findings it is perhaps not surprising that CPNs appear significantly more satisfied with their work than WBPNs.

Comparisons of the use of coping strategies revealed little difference between the two nursing groups although CPNs felt their line managers to be significantly less supportive than the hospital nurses. The use of coping strategies proved significantly effective for the ward based psychiatric nurses in increasing their sense of personal accomplishment with their work. The level of emotional exhaustion expressed by WBPNs was most effectively reduced by means of social support, the source of which could be both professional and personal, while involvement or submerging oneself in one's work appeared related to positive general health.

REFERENCES

Brown, D., Leary, J., Bartlett, H., Fagin, L. and Carson, J. (1994) Stress in the Community Psychiatric Nurse: The development of a measure. *Journal of Psychiatric and Mental Health Nursing* (submitted).

Cooper, C.L., Sloan, J.M. and Williams, S. (1988) *Occupational Stress Indicator Management Guide*, NFER-Nelson, Windsor.

Goldberg, D. and Williams, P. (1988) *A User's Guide to the General Health Questionnaire*, NFER-Nelson, Windsor.

Koelbel, P., Fuller, F. and Misener, T. (1991) Job satisfaction of nurse practitioners: an analysis using Herzberg's theory. *Nurse Practitioner,* **16**(4), 43–6.

Maslach, C. and Jackson, S. (1986) *Maslach Burnout Inventory,* Consulting Psychologists Press, California.

Rosenberg, M. (1965) *Society and the Adolescent Self-image,* Princeton University Press, Princeton, New Jersey.

CHAPTER 7

Findings from the Claybury study for community psychiatric nurses

Daniel Brown and John Leary

INTRODUCTION

Journeying between Colchester, Mile End, Canvey Island, Woodford and Chelmsford, the scale of the huge North East Thames CPN catchment area became apparent. Visiting all 15 of these departments – sometimes themselves internally geographically split – for assessment, feedback and qualitative interviews required considerable preparation, planning and travel. CPNs greatly facilitated this process and were without exception extremely courteous – countless cups of coffee were provided to the reseacher.

The CPN departments were in all cases helpful in completing lengthy questionnaires. Participants were insightful and enthusiastic about the project. CPNs were particularly interested in the feedback sessions and the discussions were thoughtful, open, illuminating and provoking. The impression gained was that CPNs are deeply concerned about and wish to contribute to the future of their rapidly expanding profession.

In this chapter we examine the results of the quantitative scores obtained by CPNs participating in the Claybury CPN Stress Study. Firstly, we cover the demographic characteristics of the group. We proceed to the essential results of the indicators used, then explore some of these results in more detail. We study how coping skills are used and how they affect stress. The CPN Stress Questionnaire is partitioned into groups of high and low scores and analysed in terms of the other stress indicators. It is further examined by ranking individual items and by factor analysis. We explore the health patterns of CPNs in terms of smoking and drinking habits. Stepwise regression is performed on both the CPN Stress Questionnaire and the General

Health Questionnaire. Finally, we offer some conclusions on the results.

METHODOLOGY

250 qualified CPNs were surveyed from 15 districts in the North East Thames Region. The researcher visited all the districts in person, administering a range of questionnaires. A standardized outline of the research project and its aims was given. Participants were assured as to the confidentiality of their questionnaires and were given as long as they wished to answer the questionnaires. The completed questionnaires were collected and marked and feedback sessions were convened where results were fed back to participants, both individually (feedback sheets) and on a group level (written report and presentation). Qualitative assessments were also administered. These are discussed in Chapter 8.

The following assessment tools were used:

1. Demographic questionnaire (see Appendix);
2. General Health Questionnaire GHQ-28 (Goldberg and Williams, 1988);
3. Maslach Burnout Inventory (Maslach and Jackson, 1986);
4. Rosenberg Self-Attitude Scale (Rosenberg, 1965);
5. Minnesota Job Satisfaction Scale (Koelbel *et al.*, 1991);
6. Coping Skills Questionnaire (Cooper *et al.*, 1988);
7. CPN Stress Questionnaire (revised) (Carson *et al.*, 1991).

RESULTS

Demographic

The average age of the sample was 39 years. Sixty two percent of the CPNs were women, 74% of the sample were married or living with a partner and 54% had children (there were 14 single parents: four men and ten women). The average annual absence was 7.2 days. Sixty five percent of CPNs felt 'happy' or 'very happy' in answer to a simple feelings question (see Appendix), whilst 8% of CPNs felt unhappy or worse. Sixty six percent of CPNs rated their fitness as good or excellent, 27% of the sample smoked and 6% smoked more than 20 cigarettes a day. Nineteen percent of CPNs drank up to or more than three units per day (one unit equals half a pint of beer). In reply to the question 'Do you have job security?', 52% of CPNs felt that they did not have job security.

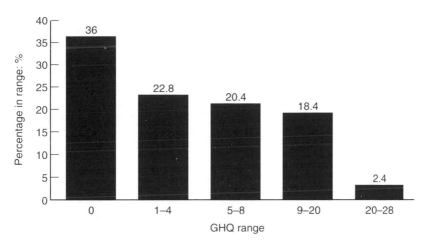

Figure 7.1 Percentage of CPNs in specified GHQ ranges.

General Health Questionnaire

We used the GHQ-28. While this version has four subscales, in non-clinical samples scores are often so low that the most appropriate indices to use were GHQ total score and percentage of psychiatric 'cases'. A level of 'psychiatric caseness' as defined by the GHQ is a score of five or more.

The average GHQ score was 4.8 (SD 5.8, range 0–27). Differences between districts were not statistically significant. However, it is worth noting that for five out of 15 departments, the average departmental score exceeds the threshold psychiatric caseness level.

Graphical presentation of the results (Figure 7.1) shows clearly that 36% of CPNs scored a healthy zero on the General Health Questionnaire. A further 22.8% of the participants were below the threshold level of 'psychiatric caseness'. However, a similar number of CPNs, 20.4%, were in the 5–8 range exceeding this threshold point, 18.4% of the sample were scoring quite highly on the GHQ and 2.4% of CPNs were at a chronic level of stress symptoms.

It can be seen that 41% of the CPNs in the sample crossed the threshold of 'psychiatric caseness' on the GHQ, scoring five or above.

Maslach Burnout Inventory

The Maslach Burnout Inventory was used to obtain an average score on each dimension of emotional exhaustion, depersonalization and personal accomplishment. The Maslach Burnout scores were compared with normative scores for the relevant occupational subgroup of mental health workers (Maslach and Jackson, 1986). Scores were then categorized as high, moderate and low burnout. The following average component scores were obtained:

Emotional exhaustion

This looks at the long-term emotional effects of stress.

Average score for CPNs: 21.5 (SD 11.5, range 0–52). This average score was in the high burnout category and 48% of CPNs scored in this category.

Depersonalization

This is a measure of how well nurses are relating to their clients.

Average score for CPNs: 5.4 (SD 5.3, range 0–25). This average score was in the moderate burnout category and 24% of CPNs scored in the high burnout category.

Personal accomplishment

This measures personal effectiveness in the work role and can be seen as an index of job satisfaction, as how much people are achieving at work.

Average score for CPNs: 34.4 (SD 7.3, range 9–48). This average score was in the low burnout category and 20% of CPNs scored in the high burnout category.

From these results, we can see that CPNs are suffering from high burnout in emotional exhaustion, but low burnout in personal accomplishment and do not feel a sense of hopelessness and futility that is commonly associated with it. However, CPNs are showing moderate depersonalization burnout levels in terms of empathizing with clients.

Rosenberg Self-Attitude Questionnaire

We used the modified version (Wycherley, 1987). Scores vary between 10 and 40 and low scores indicate better self-esteem.

Average score for CPNs: 16.6 (SD 4.7, range 10–29). This falls in the 17–20 category:

> You have an average fairly balanced view of yourself as having both good and bad points. You feel you can hold your own in comparison with others and that other people see you as neither better or worse than they are.
>
> (Wycherley, 1987)

Minnesota Job Satisfaction Scale

The scale comprises a total score indicating a level of overall job satisfaction and subscales representing intrinsic satisfaction to do with the job itself (achievement, recognition, responsibility) and extrinsic factors (salary, status, supervision).

Higher scores indicate greater job satisfaction. The scores are the total average scores for all 250 participants.

Total job satisfaction for CPNs: 66.1 (SD 10.2, range 22–93). Intrinsic job satisfaction for CPNS: 44.1 (SD 6.4, range 19–69). Extrinsic job satisfaction for CPNs: 16.4 (SD 4.6, range 6–46).

Coping skills results

The Coping Skills Questionnire taken from Cooper's Occupational Stress Indicator provides information on six types of coping strategy. These are social support (help from peers), task strategies (ways of organizing work), logic (using a detached approach), home and work relationships, time (awareness and management) and involvement (identification with work aims). The scores obtained are shown in Table 7.1. They are listed alongside the normative scores from the indicator.

Table 7.1 Comparison of CPNs use of coping strategies with normative values

Coping strategy	CPNs	Norms	% above norm range
Social support	18	9–18	45
Task strategies	26.7	17–24	72.7
Logic	12.1	10–14	9.6
Home & work relationships	17.9	10–19	35
Time management	15.3	12–17	14.1
Involvement	24.7	14–22	76.8

It can be seen that the average use of task strategies and involvement (and social support borderline) as coping strategies were higher than the normative scores. However, in investigating these scores, we must bear in mind that Cooper's mean scores were derived from studies conducted solely on British business managers.

72.7% of CPNs exceeded the normative usage for task strategies and 77% used involvement more than the norm. Social support was used more frequently than the norm by 45% of the CPNs in the sample. We split the sample according to each of these three coping strategies, testing the sector of the sample that exceeded the normative range against the sector of the sample beneath this maximum point. The following statistically significant differences were found.

For all cases of social support, task strategies and involvement coping strategies, highly significant differences were associated with all of the six coping strategies with the sole exception of social support. In this case there was no significant difference observed between high and lower usage of social support for logic as a coping strategy. This might be explained by assuming that social support is an emotional form of support, antithetical to a logical approach.

Social support

Social support was associated with increased intrinsic job satisfaction ($p < .004$) and total job satisfaction, but not extrinsic satisfaction. Better self-attitude ($p < .01$) was found for those using more social support. Strangely, CPNs using more social support had significantly lower client caseloads. This might be a reflection on the kinds of patients seen: qualitative reports noted that type and not number of clients was the determining stress factor.

Table 7.2 Differences between high and low users of social support as a means of coping for CPNs

Indicator	Lots of social support	Less social support	Significance*
Intrinsic job satisfaction	45.4	42.8	0.004
Maslach emotional exhaustion	20.2	23.1	0.04
Number of patients	31.4	36.2	0.02
Self-attitude	15.9	17.4	0.01
Age	37.9	40.5	0.01
Years	14.6	16.5	0.02

*Mann-Whitney test

Interestingly, social support is used more on average by people of a lower age group and those who have been fewer years in the same job. High levels of social support showed no significant differences on the General Health Questionnaire. However, the long-term emotional exhaustion effects were significantly lower with greater levels of social support ($p < 0.04$).

Task strategies

A different pattern emerged for task strategy coping. Client caseload numbers were significantly different for task strategies, but in the opposite direction than for social support. Greater use of task strategy was associated with greater numbers of patients. It may be that handling larger numbers of clients requires more efficient task strategies. CPNs working with a specific client group were more likely to use more task strategy coping than those not working with a specific client group. GHQ scores were significantly lower when more task strategy coping was used. Long-term emotional exhaustion burnout was greatly reduced, showing a highly significant difference (p<.00001) when high levels of task strategy coping were utilized. Again, intrinsic and total job satisfaction were greater when more task strategies were used. However, task strategy was also associated with improved extrinsic job satisfaction (pay, status, etc.). Stereotypically, gender differences were associated with task strategies. A greater percentage of male CPNs used high levels of task strategy coping than female CPNs.

Table 7.3 Differences between high and low users of task strategies as a means of coping for CPNs

Indicator	Lots of task strategy	Less task strategy	Significance*
GHQ	3.6	5.3	0.03
Intrinsic job satisfaction	44.5	42.5	0.02
Extrinsic job satisfaction	16.8	15	0.02
Maslach emotional exhaustion	19.8	27.1	0.00001
Number of patients	35.1	31.2	0.02
Self-attitude	16.3	17.9	0.03
Group	1.26	1.4	0.05
Sex	1.57	1.72	0.05

*Mann-Whitney test

Involvement

Greater levels of involvement were again associated with increased intrinsic and total job satisfaction, but not with extrinsic job satisfaction. GHQ levels were lower with more involvement. Long-term burnout effects in emotional exhaustion were not associated with involvement as a coping strategy. However, personal accomplishment

Table 7.4 Differences between high and low users of involvement as a means of coping for CPNs

Indicator	Lots of involvement	Less involvement	Significance*
Absence	5.8	12.4	0.03
Fitness	2.2	2.5	0.001
GHQ	5.7	3.5	0.03
Intrinsic job satisfaction	44.4	42.6	0.03
Maslach personal accomplishment	35	32.1	0.02

*Mann-Whitney test

burnout (feelings of hopelessness and futility) were significantly lower with more involvement – on this scale numerically higher scores indicate lower burnout. Fitness was substantially greater for those using more involvement as a coping strategy (p<.001). It may be that those more involved in their work are exercising more.

Greater use of involvement as a coping strategy was associated with significantly fewer days absence – 5.8 days for those using high levels of involvement compared with 12.4 days in general.

CPN Stress Questionnaire (Revised)

This 48-item questionnaire was developed by us at Claybury hospital specifically for investigating the causes of stress for CPNs. An original 66-item questionnaire using a 0–4 Likert scale was developed from examining available literature and interviewing CPNs from four districts and compiling a list of stressors. The resulting questionnaire was then reduced to 48 items through item discrimination and correlation analyses. The instrument has been shown to be split half and test–retest reliable and to have concurrent and construct validity (Brown *et al.*, 1994).

The average CPN Stress Questionnaire was 78.0 (SD 29.6, range 13–161). There was no significant difference (ANOVA analysis) between departments.

Comparison of high and low stress groups

We wished to examine the effect of high stress levels at work. The results of the CPN Stress Questionnaire from the total sample of 250 approximated a normal distribution. We partitioned the results of the lower third of the scores and the upper third of the scores and

Table 7.5 Comparison of high and low stress scorers on the CPN stress questionnaire

Indicator	CPN low	CPN high
GHQ	2.5	7.7
Maslach emotional exhaustion	14.5	28.8
Maslach depersonalization	3.3	7.2
Maslach personal accomplishment	36.6	32.5
Job satisfaction	70	62.3
Self-attitude	15.3	17.7
Attitude of line manager	1.9	2.2
Job security	1.4	1.7
Number of patients	30.1	35
Absence (days)	4.8	11.1

compared these two groups to see if there were statistically significant differences between them on a range of measures including demographic and the test instruments (1–6). We found statistically significant differences as shown in Table 7.5.

GHQ, Maslach emotional exhaustion and depersonalization scores were, as we might expect, higher for high stressor levels – assuming the CPN Stress Questionnaire score approximates to a measure of perceived stress. The attitude of the line manager was perceived as significantly worse for those experiencing higher levels of stress. Self-esteem was significantly lower for those experiencing greater stress.

There was a significant difference in days absent – this amounted on average to six days annually between the higher and lower stress groups. These results indicate very concrete sequelae of stress, contradicting critics of the applicability of the concept of stress (e.g. Briner and Reynolds, 1993). Whilst qualitative research showed that type and not number of patients was the stress determining factor, the number of patients does seem quantitatively important: the high stress group averaged five more patients than the lower stress group.

We noted that none of the coping skills showed statistically significant differences between the high and low stressor groups.

Job satisfaction was greater for those experiencing less stress. Since higher scores on personal accomplishment show lower burnout, the low CPN stress score group indicated greater feelings of personal accomplishment than the high CPN stress group.

We cannot say with certainty what causes what – for example, whether higher stress causes a worse relationship with the line manager or attribution of a bad relationship with a line manager through transference or whether higher stress is an effect of a poor relationship with a line manager. As was discussed in an earlier chapter, we have found the causes and effects of stress to be closely inter-related and often inseparable. All we can conclude is that there is some statistically significant correlation between high stress levels in CPNs and the quality of the relationship with the line manager. And this is the same with all of the 'cause–effect' relationships.

Analysis by item ranking

The results from all 48 items on the 250 completed CPN Stress Questionnaires were analysed by ranking the overall average value of the Likert (0–4) score for each item. The ten most and least stressful items were then listed as shown in Table 7.6.

Table 7.6 Item rankings: the ten least stressful items – rated by CPNs on the Stress Questionnaire

Rank	Ten least stressful items	Mean stress score range (0–4)
1	Having to carry drugs around	0.84
2	Not feeling you can rely on the support of CPN colleagues	1.01
3	Having to drive a lot in the course of a week	1.16
4	Feeling there is a communication problem with CPN colleagues	1.2
5	Having to obtain a suitable caseload/experience for students	1.31
6	Having to cope with changes in the job	1.31
7	Having to work in isolation	1.32
8	Having to receive supervision you do not find helpful	1.35
9	Having problems getting to some clients' homes	1.36
10	Having to put up with interruptions when seeing clients at home	1.38

Many of these items would be expected to fall into the least stressful categories. Having to carry drugs around is unlikely to cause any difficulties for an experienced psychiatric nurse. Having to drive a lot and working in isolation appear to be acceptable parts of a CPN's job.

Likewise, getting to clients' homes and having to put up with interruptions when seeing clients at home are an accepted part of the work. Having to obtain a suitable caseload for students does not seem to have inconvenienced too many CPNs.

Some of the results emerging from the list of least stressful items are encouraging. (2) 'Not feeling that I can rely on the support of CPN colleagues' and (4) 'Feeling that there is a communication problem with CPN colleagues' indicates that on balance CPNs are supportive and communicating well with each other. Because (8) 'Having to receive supervision that you do not find helpful' is among the least stressful items, we can assume that in fact supervisions are helpful for CPNs and indeed this was confirmed in the qualitative part of the research. However, management communication does not occupy any of the ten least stressful slots and this is of concern.

Table 7.7 item rankings: the ten most stressful items – rated by CPNs on the Stress Questionnaire

Rank	Ten most stressful items	Mean stress score (range 0–4)
1	Not having facilities in the community that you can refer clients onto	2.38
2	Knowing there are likely to be long waiting lists before clients can get access to services	2.17
3	Having to deal with suicidal clients on your own	2.17
4	Not having enough time for study or personal improvement	2.12
5	Trying to keep up a good quality of care in your work	2.1
6	Having too many interruptions when trying to work in the office	2.08
7	Having to visit unsafe areas	2.06
8	Feeling there is not enough hospital back-up	1.98
9	Having to work with clients with a known history of violence	1.97
10	Having to cope with changes at your workbase	1.93

The top two most stressful items – 'Not having facilities that you can refer clients onto' and 'Knowing there are likely to be long waiting lists before clients can get access to services – were both centred on a lack of facilities. It is ironic to note the conflict of our results with the government White Paper Caring For People (DoH, 1989) which reports that 'As community workers, nurses are in close touch with the network of help available in a neighbourhood and can mobilize resources to respond sensitively to people's needs'.

Safety issues were also causing stress. Thus (3) 'Having to deal with suicidal clients on your own', (7) 'Having to visit unsafe areas' and (9) 'Having to work with clients with a known history of violence' indicate that there are real safety problems for psychiatric nurses working in the community.

Office problems are highly stressful: (7) 'Having too many interruptions when trying to work in the office' and (10) 'Having to cope with changes at your workbase express some of the simple practical difficulties that can have significant adverse effects on the working day of a CPN.

While (5) 'Trying to keep up a good quality of care in your work' appears innocuous, it is ranked the fifth most stressful item. It may be at the heart of many other stress problems experienced by CPNs. In an earlier chapter, we mentioned the working definition of stress as the external demands of the situation against the internal resources to cope with them. It appears that CPNs have substantial demands placed upon them, with inadequate back-up and resources. When that is coupled with a desire to provide a good quality of care, which it is impossible to provide, this makes life very stressful. The question then is: should CPNs accept that they often cannot give a good quality of care to patients, which would decrease stress levels but decrease the efforts for patient care, or should they continue to attempt to provide a good quality of care with all the personal stress that this produces?

Health patterns

Sixty six per cent of the CPNs rated their fitness as good or excellent. Smoking and drinking patterns are alternatively viewed as coping strategies or symptomatic stress responses. We looked at the smoking and drinking patterns of the sample with reference to the stress patterns.

Smoking

Twenty seven per cent of the CPNs in our sample were smokers and 6% smoked more than 20 cigarettes per day. A detailed analysis of smokers (27%) and non-smokers (73%) in the sample investigated whether there were significant stress differences between those who did smoke and those who did not smoke. The results obtained are shown in Table 7.8.

CPN smokers averaged significantly higher emotional exhaustion than non-smokers ($p < .02$), a difference that represented a transition

Table 7.8 Significant differences between CPN smokers and non-smokers

Type	Av. non-smoker	Av. smoker	Significance*
Emotional exhaustion	20.4	24.6	0.02
Depersonalization	4.9	6.7	0.01
GHQ	4.3	6.2	0.02
Self-attitude	16	18.3	0.001
Annual days absence	6.2	10.1	0.05
Alcohol	2.98	2.69	0.001
Children	1.41	1.57	0.05
Feel	3.75	3.45	0.02
Fitness	2.2	2.46	0.05

*Mann-Whitney test

between moderate and high burnout on the Maslach normative values for mental health workers. Likewise there were significant differences in depersonalization – smokers had on average significantly lower empathy for clients ($p<.01$). Smokers had significantly higher GHQ scores ($p<.02$) and felt unhappier on the simple FEEL measure ('How do you feel about your life as a whole at the moment?' – see Appendix). On average, smokers were above the threshold level of psychiatric caseness, while non-smokers were on average below this level. Smokers were found to have a poorer self-attitude than non-smokers ($p<.001$). Smokers were found on average to feel less fit ($p<.05$), drink more alcohol ($p<.001$) and to take four more days absence per year ($p<.05$) than non-smokers. Non-smokers were significantly more likely to have children than were smokers ($p<.05$). There were no significant age or gender differences found between CPN smokers and non-smokers.

Scores in personal accomplishment, the CPN Stress Questionnaire and job satisfaction scores were not found to be significantly different for smokers and non-smokers.

We noted that it is hard to postulate a causal relationship: are smokers absent more because they are less fit as a consequence of smoking or because stress pressures are directly causing illness or exhaustion? We can say, however, that higher emotional exhaustion is associated with higher levels of smoking and this is a health concern.

Alcohol consumption

We compared the CPN sample for those people who drank up to three units per day or more than three units per day (19%) and those who drank only occasionally or never (81%). The only significant differences between the two groups are shown in Table 7.9.

Table 7.9 Significant differences between CPNs drinking more and less

Type	Av. drink more	Av. drink less	Significance*
GHQ	6.8	4.3	0.04
Children	1.58	1.43	0.05
Cigarettes	1.91	1.42	0.0007
Sex	1.45	1.66	.01

*Mann-Whitney test

CPNs drinking more were found to have significantly higher GHQ scores than those drinking less. However, there were no significant differences found on any of the long-term burnout scores for heavier and occasional drinkers. CPNs drinking more were significantly more likely not to have children than those drinking less. Higher levels of drinking were associated with higher smoking levels. Unlike the findings for smokers, there was a significant gender difference associated with drinking habits: heavier drinkers were significantly more likely to be men.

These findings suggest that drinking and smoking habits are related to stress experiences at work. Smoking was associated with more of the measures than drinking and there was an association between perceived fitness and smoking levels, which did not occur with drinking patterns. Both habits were, however, linked with the GHQ and with each other. The levels of cigarette smoking suggest that stress levels may be having an adverse effect on the health of the CPNs. It may be that smoking is regarded as a coping strategy or that coping simply increases when people are agitated. It is noteworthy that statistically smokers have a lower self-attitude than non-smokers, as measured on the Rosenberg Self-Attitude Scale. This was not found to be the case with the drinking comparison groups.

Factor analysis

All the 48 items in the CPN Stress Questionnaire were factor analysed for the total sample of CPNs. The following five factors accounted for 51.7% of the total variance and are thus considered as key groupings of stress issues for CPNs (items within the factors were included at a factor loading $p > 0.5$):

Factor 1 (29.8 of total variance): support and communication

30. Not feeling that I have sufficient support from my line manager.
31. Feeling that I can rely on the support of my CPN colleagues.
32. Feeling that the management style within our department is inflexible.
33. Feeling that there is a lack of communication with management.
34. Feeling there is a communication problem with my CPN colleagues.
35. Not having enough internal supervision within the department.
36. Having to receive supervision that I do not find helpful.
37. Feeling that other people underestimate my skills as a CPN.

Factor 2 (7.3% of total variance): safety issues

22. Having to visit unsafe areas.
23. Having to carry drugs around.
24. Having to work with clients with a known history of violence.
25. Having to deal with suicidal clients on my own.
26. Trying to maintain therapeutic control in the client's home.

Factor 3 (6.1% of the total variance): perceived CPN role

12. Feeling that my role as a CPN is misunderstood by other professionals.
13. Feeling that other people expect too much from me as a CPN.
14. Not being shown sufficient respect by other professionals.
15. Not getting the proper amount of co operation from other health workers.
16. Having communication problems with other professionals.

Factor 4 (4.4% of total variance): therapeutic client work

38. Having to work with clients that are unco-operative.
39. Working with clients that I don't particularly like.
40. Having to work with resistive couples or families.
41. Having to put up with interruptions when seeing clients at home.

Factor 5 (4.1% of total variance): problems of referral

17. Having to see inappropriate referrals.
18. Receiving referrals that are incomplete.
19. Not being informed of treatment changes affecting my client.
20. Having to do things for my clients which I don't feel are part of a CPN's job.

Clearly support and communication are the key variant factors moderating stress for CPNs, Safety issues are also a major concern. The changing role of a CPN is particularly stressful in light of its perception by other mental health workers. Problems of referral are a significant source of variance and these may be connected to perceived CPN roles in subtle ways. From the factor analysis, we also conclude that issues of actual client work are important in determining CPN stress levels. These five factors accorded largely with research previously conducted in a Q sort analysis (Leary *et al.*, 1994).

Regression analysis

A stepwise linear regression analysis was conducted, using both the CPN Stress Questionnaire and GHQ results as the dependent variables. The CPN Stress Questionnaire analysis was completed in two ways. Firstly, we examined only demographic data to look at the predictive scope of these demographic factors. An equation was obtained with an R square value of 10%:

Demographic predictors of high CPN stress scores

The stepwise multiple regression analysis indicated that four variables were the best predictors of CPN stress scores for CPNs. The overall R square of the equation was 10%. The four predicting variables were:

1. happiness with present life;
2. number of patients;
3. absence;
4. relationship with line manager.

1. The unhappier people were, the higher the stress score.
2. The higher the number of patients, the greater the CPN stress score. Interestingly, there is no question on the CPN Stress Questionnaire which asks the number of patients the CPN is seeing – this figure is on the demographic questionnaire. The number of patients may therefore have an effect, for example, on the perceived support of management – or vice versa. Furthermore, in qualitative research, CPNs have commented that it is the type and not the quantity of patients that affects stress levels. However, this regression result and the previous analysis of high and low stress scores suggests that quantity of patients does determine stress levels
3. There was a linear relationship between annual days off absent and the CPN Stress Questionnaire, such that increased absence levels were associated with high stress scores.

4. The worse the relationship with the line manager, the higher the stress levels on the CPN Stress Questionnaire.

General predictors of high CPN Stress Questionnaire scores

When we included all the possible variables of the other psychometric instruments in the stepwise regression equation, the R squared value was 34%.

The five predictive variables were:

1. Maslach emotional exhaustion;
2. extrinsic job satisfaction;
3. intrinsic job satisfaction;
4. task strategy coping;
5. Maslach personal accomplishment.

1. High Maslach emotional exhaustion scores predicted high CPN Stress Questionnaire scores.
2. There was a negative relation to the CPN Stress Questionnaire Score: the higher the satisfaction, the lower the stress.
3. Contrary to the previous relationship, the higher the satisfaction on the actual job, the higher the stress. This at first seems contrary to expectations. However, the coping strategies analysis may provide some explanation. The analysis showed that the involvement coping strategy is greatly used by CPNs. Immersion in work may be more satisfying but it is also likely to generate more stress.
4. The more frequently the task strategy coping measure was used, the higher the CPN Stress Questionnaire Score. Whilst we can observe that there is an increased use of coping strategy, we cannot from this regression analysis determine whether there is a corresponding effect in reducing the stress levels. However, from the coping skills analysis (see p. 124), we did find that the group using more task strategies had lower emotional exhaustion burnout levels (yet not significantly lower CPN Stress Questionnaire levels) than a group using fewer task strategies.
5. The Maslach personal accomplishment variable had a negative relation to CPN stress scores. Low burnout (i.e. high numerical scores) predicts lower CPN Stress Questionnaire scores. As we might expect, feelings of personal accomplishment have a positive effect on reducing CPN stress scores. This positive effect is a crucial mediator in stress levels.

Predictors of high GHQ scores

We further performed a stepwise regression analysis on the GHQ scores. Here all potential demographic indicators were entered into the analysis. The R squared value was 53%.

The six predictive variables were:

1. Maslach emotional exhaustion;
2. fitness;
3. happiness;
4. CPN stress score;
5. self-attitude;
6. ENB.

1. High levels of emotional exhaustion burnout predicted high GHQ scores.
2. Lower levels of fitness were linked with lower GHQ. This is interesting because the GHQ contains no direct reference to physical fitness, it focuses on symptoms of stress such as restlessness and poor concentration.
3. Unhappiness predicted high GHQ scores.Thus both physical fitness and emotional feelings contribute to the GHQ score.
4. Whilst the GHQ score did not show up in the regression analysis of the CPN Stress Questionnaire as dependent variable, CPN stress is a contributing factor to the GHQ score when the GHQ is the dependent variable. As we would expect, the higher the level of perceived stressors measured on the CPN Stress Questionnaire, the higher the GHQ score.
5. Poor self-attitude predicted higher GHQ scores.
6. The question: 'Have you completed the specialist ENB course in community psychiatric nursing? (1=yes, 2=no, see Appendix) indicated that not having an ENB is predictive of higher GHQ scores.

It is interesting that with GHQ as dependent variable, the CPN stress score entered into the equation, whilst GHQ did not enter the CPN stress score equation. This might be expected because the CPN Stress Questionnaire looked more at stressors than the GHQ which examined stress symptoms, of which the stressors would be a cause.

CONCLUSIONS

Overall, we conclude that CPNs are experiencing high levels of stress. The GHQ indicates that 41% of CPNs have crossed a threshold level of so-called psychiatric caseness. This does not necessarily mean that 41% of CPNs are on a borderline of breakdown, but it does imply that all is not well within the profession. Measured against a normative sample of mental health workers, 48% of CPNs were experiencing high levels of long-term emotional exhaustion burnout. Twenty four

per cent of CPNs were suffering from high levels of depersonalization burnout and not relating well to clients while 20% of CPNs were
experiencing severe long-term feelings of lack of personal accomplishment at work.

We found CPNs to have a healthy self-attitude: the average score
indicated CPNs to have 'a fairly well balanced view of self, encompassing both good and bad points', according to normative scores on
the Rosenberg Self-Attitude Questionnaire.

CPNs were obtaining overall satisfaction from their jobs, despite
the toll of stress and burnout. On average, most CPNs were satisfied
by the intrinsic factors of actual work, but not by the surrounding work
conditions – the extrinsic factors of the job.

For coping strategies, CPNs relied most on involvement task
strategies and social support. These all scored above the normative
range indicated on the Cooper questionnaire, although these normative
scores were restricted to British business managers only. Greater use
of all three strategies was associated with greater overall job satisfaction. However, only task strategies correlated with higher extrinsic
job satisfaction.

GHQ scores were lower with greater use of involvement and task
strategies. Long-term emotional exhaustion was significantly reduced
with greater use of task strategies and social support. Self-attitude
was better for those using more social support (p<.01) and task
strategies (p<.03) but not involvement. Greater involvement was
associated with considerably reduced absenteeism (5.8 days) compared
with lower levels of involvement (12.4 days). This might be useful
to bear in mind when managing and motivating a CPN team.

Older people used social support less than younger people. Those
who had spent longer in their jobs also used social support less than
those newer to their jobs. People who have been employed in a job
a long time could benefit from training groups (see Carson, 1994).

The absence rate varied directly with the level of stress. We found
that CPNs experiencing more stress took more time off (the top third
most stressed averaged 11.1 days) than CPNs experiencing less stress
(the bottom third least stressed averaged 4.8 days).

That high CPN Stress Questionnaire, high GHQ and high Maslach
Burnout Inventory Scores were related was as predicted (Brown *et
al.*, 1994). We found a significant difference of six days per year absence
between the top third most stressed and bottom third least stressed
CPNs as measured on the CPN Stress Questionnaire. Whilst qualitative
research indicated that type and not number of patients was the stress
determining factor, the number of patients does seem quantitatively
important: the high stress group averaged five more patients than the
lower stress group. Reducing client caseload levels would seem to be
a priority for reducing stress levels.

Smokers averaged significantly higher GHQ and emotional exhaustion scores yet stressors as measured on the CPN Stress Questionnaire showed no significant differences between smokers and non-smokers. Smokers took four more days off per year than non-smokers on average and also had a significantly poorer self-attitude. High levels of smoking and drinking were correlated. Heavy drinking was associated with higher GHQ scores, but not with long-term burnout.

From the rankings of the CPN Stress Questionnaire, the least stressful items indicated that on balance CPNs were supportive and communicating well with each other and were receiving helpful supervisions. The most stressful items indicated that lack of facilities in the community and long referral waiting lists were the two most stressful issues for CPNs. Safety issues of dealing with violent and suicidal clients and having to visit unsafe areas were also very stressful. Office problems of interruptions in the office and coping with changes in the workbase were also causing stress. Added to this, the aims and efforts of CPNs to provide a good quality of care against the obstacles set against them was causing a high level of stress in itself.

The factor analysis largely concorded with earlier research completed in a Q sort analysis in producing similar factors (Leary *et al.*, 1994). The five factors obtained demonstrate concisely some major concerns of CPNs. Key moderating factors producing a variance in stress levels were found to be:

1. support and communication from management and colleagues;
2. safety issues;
3. perceived CPN role.

The regression analysis identified that GHQ scores were predicted by fitness, happiness, emotional exhaustion, self-attitude and the CPN Stress Questionnaire score (which might be said to approximate to an indicator of stressors). The CPN Stress Questionnaire itself was predicted by task strategy coping, personal accomplishment, job satisfaction and emotional exhaustion and by demographic factors of numbers of patients, happiness and relationship with line manager. Particularly important was that personal accomplishment and extrinsic job satisfaction were predictive of lowering the perceived stressors. This could be borne in mind by management.

It is clearly essential, given the high levels of stress that we have found in our study of CPNs, to find methods of reducing these stress levels. Approaches may focus directly on the symptoms of stress (both immediate and long-term burnout) such as relaxation exercises. They may address the way that CPNs respond to stressful situations through supervision and support groups or individual psychotherapies looking at coping strategies and self-attitude. They may be practical methods at work, ranging from simply changing the layout of an office to reduce the number of interruptions at work to arranging with a colleague to visit a dangerous client in a pair. They may involve improving manageral practice and communication – both from the perspective of manager and managed. They may involve some forms of political action to lower the level of client caseload. We address such approaches in following chapters.

Key findings

- 41% of CPNs crossed the threshold level of GHQ caseness.
- 48% of CPNs were experiencing high levels of long-term emotional burnout.
- CPNs identified the most stressful issues as:

  1. lack of referral facilities in the community, long waiting lists for client services and lack of hospital back-up;
  2. safety issues in dealing with violent and suicidal clients;
  3. problems with the place of work.

- Factor analysis identified the key mediating factor (30% of total variance) for reducing stress as support and communication from managers and colleagues.
- Long-term emotional exhaustion was significantly lower with greater use of involvement and social support coping strategies. GHQ scores were significantly lower with greater use of involvement and task strategies.
- There was a significant difference of six days per year absence between the top third most stressed and the bottom third least stressed CPNs as measured on the CPN Stress Questionnaire. The high stress group averaged five more patients than the low stress group: reducing client case levels appears to be a priority.
- Predictors of stress symptoms were:

  1. long-term emotional burnout;
  2. fitness;
  3. feelings of happiness/unhappiness;
  4. self-esteem;
  5. having ENB training.

- Smokers averaged significantly higher GHQ and emotional exhaustion scores yet stressors as measured on the CPN Stress Questionnaire showed no significant differences between smokers and non-smokers. Smokers took four more days off per year than non-smokers on average.

Appendix

CLAYBURY CPN STRESS STUDY

DEMOGRAPHIC DATA SHEET (CPNs)

Research Number:

The following questions are designed to give us background material for the study. Your answers to this and all questionnaires will remain anonymous and strictly confidential. Please answer all the questions. The questions require you to write your answers or to circle the appropriate number.

1. Please give your age ---------------- years.

2. Sex: Male   1
          Female 2

3. Please indicate your current marital status:

    Married/living with partner   1
    Not married/separated   2

4. Do you have children living at home?

    Yes 1
    No   2

5. What is your current nursing grade (circle one)?

    A   B   C   D   E   F   G   H   I

6. Do you work with a specific group e.g. elderly?

    Yes 1
    No   2

    If so which one --------------------------------

7. Do you have an RMN?

    Yes 1
    No   2

8. Have you completed the specialist ENB course in community psychiatric nursing?

    Yes 1
    No   2

9. Do you have any additional nursing qualifications e.g. RGN?

    Yes 1
    No   2

    Please list these -------------------------------------

10. How many years have you worked in psychiatric nursing (including your training)?

---------------------- ----------- years

11. How do you rate your current level of fitness?

Excellent   1
Good   2
Fair   3
Poor   4

12. How much alcohol do you consume?

(One unit = half a pint of beer or a standard measure of spirits or one glass of wine)

Three or more units every day   1
Up to three units/day on average   2
Occasionally   3
Never drink alcohol   4

13. How many cigarettes do you smoke each day?

None   1
Less than 10   2
11 to 20   3
More than 20   4

14. How many days off for all types of sickness absence have you had in the past 12 months?

------------------------------ days

15. How do you feel about your life as a whole at present?

Very happy   5
Happy   4
Neither happy/unhappy   3
Unhappy   2
Very unhappy   1

16. What would you say are the three most stressful things in your job as a CPN?

1.
2.
3.

17. What would you say is the most stressful thing that has happened to you at work in the last month?

---- ------------------------------------

18. What helps you cope best with the pressures of your job?

--------- ------------------------------

19. How would you describe the attitude of your line manager towards you?

    Very supportive   1
    Supportive   2
    Not supportive   3
    Very unsupportive   4

20. Can you discuss any problems you have at work with one of your colleagues?

    Yes 1
    No   2

21. How long have you worked in your present job?

    -------------------------------- years

22. Do you feel you have good job security in your present job?

    Yes 1
    No   2

23. How many patients do you currently have on your caseload?

    ------------------------------- patients

REFERENCES

Briner, R. and Reynolds, S. (1993) *Bad Theory and Bad Practice in Occupational Stress*, Memo 1405, MRC Social and Applied Psychology Unit, University of Sheffield.

Brown, D., Leary, J., Bartlett, H., Fagin, L. and Carson, J. (1994) Stress in community psychiatric nurses: the development of a measure. *Journal of Psychiatric and Mental Health Nursing* (submitted).

Carson, J., Bartlett, H., Leary, J. and Gallagher, T. (1991) Stress in community psychiatric nursing: a preliminary investigation. *Community Psychiatric Nursing Journal*, 2, 8–13.

Carson, J. (1994) *Social Support Group Therapy – Treatment Manual*, unpublished manuscript available from the author.

Cooper, C.L., Sloan, S.J. and Williams, S. (1988) *Occupational Stress Indicator Management Guide*, NFER-Nelson, Windsor.

Department of Health (1989) *Caring for People*, HMSO, London.

Goldberg, D. and Williams, P. (1988) *A User's Guide to the General Health Questionnaire*, NFER-Nelson, Windsor.

Koelbel, P., Fuller, F. and Misener, T. (1991) Job satisfaction of nurse practitioners: an analysis using Herzberg's theory. *Nurse Practitioner* 16(4), 43–6.

Leary, J., Gallagher, T., Carson, J. *et al.* (1994) The use of Q-methodology to look at stress and coping in CPNs. *Journal of Advanced Nursing* (in press).

Maslach, C. and Jackson, S. (1986) *Maslach Burnout Inventory*, Consulting Psychologists Press, California.

Rosenberg, M. (1965) *Society and The Adolescent Self-Image*, Princeton University Press, Princeton, New Jersey.

Wycherley, B. (1987) *The Living Skills Pack*, South East Thames Regional Health Authority, Bexhill.

CHAPTER 8

Findings from the qualitative measures for CPNs

*Jerome Carson, Heather Bartlett, Daniel Brown
and Patrick Hopkinson*

In this chapter we report on the findings from the qualitative measures that we used in the Claybury CPN Stress Study. Earlier chapters (Chapters 6 and 7) have presented the main quantitative results from the study. We begin this chapter by discussing the advantages and disadvantages of qualitative methods in research of this kind. We then present three main types of qualitative data:

1. group discussions;
2. individual interviews with CPNs;
3. open-ended questions on the demographic questionnaires;

Following this, we then suggest what the implications of these findings are for CPNs.

THE MERITS OF QUALITATIVE METHODS

In devising the research protocol for the Claybury CPN Stress Study, we were heavily drawn to quantitative methods (Chapter 5). When we discussed the methodology of the study with two of the Region's research advisors, Dr Colin Sanderson and Dr Sue Beardsell, they suggested the inclusion of a qualitative dimension into the study. While quantitative methods could demonstrate that there were statistical differences between CPNs and ward based staff, they would not be so illuminating in helping us understand why such differences might exist. Qualitative methods opened up extra possibilities for us.

It would, however, be incorrect to assume that we had not considered qualitative methods ourselves. Indeed, John Leary had developed a Q sort study (Stephenson, 1936) to look at the issues of stress and coping well before we embarked on our major investigation. This Q sort study involved 44 CPNs and formed part of Tim Gallagher's BSc thesis at the University of East London (Gallagher, 1992). Just recently this work has been written up (Leary *et al.*, 1994).

A number of us found the Q sort methodology rather complex, so for our major study we decided to use a different approach. The first method we chose was to conduct group discussions with CPNs on a departmental basis. The second was to carry out intensive individual interviews with CPNs on their own. Both sets of interviews were naturally focused around the issues of stress and coping. We decided to only loosely structure these interviews, so that CPNs would basically be able to contribute their own thoughts to the discussions. We did not want to force them into a rather rigid question and answer session. We felt that by utilizing semistructured interviews and discussions we would benefit because:

1. CPNs would not be forced into responding in a particular way when answering questionnaires;
2. quantitative methods, by focusing on statistical significance levels, often lose a 'human feel' to the data;
3. CPNs might be able to provide us with invaluable insights into how they perceived their work;
4. the data obtained would be direct from 'the coal face'.

While qualitative methods have a number of advantages (Goldstein, 1993; Silverman, 1993) they can also provide the researcher with additional problems. For instance, conducting individual interviews is time consuming. We could give all the quantitative measures to a whole department of CPNs, check and collect all the questionnaires back in less than the time it takes to do one individual interview! Similarly, it is often difficult to arrange a series of individual interviews in a department, particularly when one is working under time pressure. There are also a number of methodological problems with group discussions.

Inevitably, as in most groups, discussions may be dominated by two or three more vocal members. This can make it harder for the more reserved members of staff to offer their opinions. Despite these caveats, we found group discussions to be very lively, with much debate around the general issues of stress and coping.

FINDINGS FROM THE GROUP DISCUSSIONS

Some 51 CPNs participated in group discussions. Five departments were surveyed and group size ranged from a minimum of eight members to a maximum of 12. The discussions were focused around 13 prompt questions and responses to these were transcribed by the researcher. On two occasions a second researcher was present, so the interviewer could focus entirely on the group process and not worry about recording the responses. The data will be presented in the order in which questions were asked. For some questions, responses for specific districts will be quoted verbatim, to give readers a 'feel' for the interviews. There will then be a brief summary of the responses to the questions from the other districts.

Question 1: What is most stressful in the job of a CPN?

District E

CPN 1   It's not the job itself, you can get a high out of that. It is the pressure from management, also the lack of support and help. I wish there was someone there who was taking an interest in what I was doing.

CPN 2   Managers can see you are under stress. Your team is getting smaller, yet they tell you to carry on. If your caseload is too big, they tell you to get rid of some clients.

CPN 3   A senior manager asked me, 'How many do you have on your caseload? Oh, that's too many, you'll become ill. Have you told the team leader about this?' In fact the team leader has more cases that I have!

CPN 4   I asked for a simple thing. A bleep. I do around 1000 miles a month. I had to travel back to the team base to see a client, but they weren't there. They had been trying to contact me. I had to travel 20 miles. One day something serious will happen.

CPN 5   I didn't have a desk. I sat on a chair at the back of the office. When I asked for a desk I was told, 'You're a CPN, you should be out in the community'. The social worker was on leave so I was able to use her desk.

CPN 6   (Taking up the theme of desks) I had three occupational therapists arrive in the office one day. They asked to use my desk. They had been told I only used the office and desk for one hour in the morning and the rest of the day it was free.

Summary

The above comments represent some of the statements from CPNs in one district. Broadly, responses from all districts could be categorized into five major groups.

1. Logistical problems: 'driving when the traffic is bad', 'picking up parking tickets'.
2. Perception of CPNs: 'people think all CPNs do is give injections'.
3. Liaison with other professionals.
4. The pressure of working individually in the community: 'the lack of a back-up system'.
5. Confusion around aspects of community care: 'You feel you are the key worker. But you are not sure if you have authority to co-ordinate care'.

A final comment from one CPN describes the stresses of being a CPN:

> It's the demands or needs that we cannot respond to. It feels like painting on a large canvas with a small brush. There is a huge waiting list, so much could be done if resources were there ...

Question 2: Have you found any recent incidents especially stressful?

District B

CPN 1 Yesterday was very anxiety provoking. I went to this woman's house. I'd been told by the psychiatrists she wasn't well, but the information I had was very vague, I didn't know what to expect.

CPN 2 I went to see someone in his house last night at 5 o'clock. He's a depressed client whose wife is in hospital. He says he is suicidal. He pulled out a gun. I just took the gun in my hand. I said, 'Is it loaded?'. He said, 'No'. I gave it back to him and he put it in a drawer. When I left I contacted the police. It was on my mind last night. The shock. When it happened I went into overdrive and cut off my emotions. Safety is a hot issue for us. Yet no-one knew where I was. I thought he was safe. My imagination was in riot going home. He could have shot someone!

Summary

Three main issues arose here:

1. Dealing with suicidal clients: 'I found a patient had cut her throat. I was affected for a long time and still am'.
2. The risk element of working in the community.
3. Problems with general practitioners: 'One GP treats us with contempt. Patients are sent to us with their notes in their hands'.

Question 3: How do the stresses in CPN work vary from ward work?

District C

CPN 1   On a ward there are clearer boundaries. I worry less about personal security.

CPN 2   Handing over clients so you can go on leave is difficult. It becomes hugely stressful to organize a holiday.

CPN 3   Working on the ward you get ward politics. There are conflicts that develop over people not doing things. You get that a little bit in the community, but essentially you are your own boss.

CPN 4   One rewarding thing in the community is the length of the relationship with clients. In a ward, you see someone, you start to get to know them, then they are out. It's nice to see clients when they are not disturbed.

Summary

Again, three main themes arose here:

1. Time management: 'You can't get things done fast enough'.
2. Autonomy versus isolation: 'You can't go out of the room and ask someone what to do in a situation'.
3. The nature of the therapeutic relationship. Most CPNs felt that this was a positive feature, in that they could establish longer term relationships with clients.

Question 4: Could managers help in any way to reduce stress?

District B

CPN 1   In the community we need someone to hold us together and someone with the ability to make decisions.

CPN 2   We need a structure provided. People need space to say what is difficult.

CPN 3   I think good supervision is the key. When I was in hospital I had none. It's the single most valuable thing for me. Other faults go away if there's good supervision.

CPN 4   In this particular service there does not seem to be a vision of how the service will develop. Managers should provide that. Similarly there is a lack of idea how to deliver a service in the community.

Summary

CPNs were not reticent in offering ideas about how managers could reduce their work stress.

1. Be more understanding.
2. Provide better facilities for CPNs, 'office space and secretarial support'.
3. Allow greater involvement in decision making and planning.

Question 5: How do you cope with the pressures of your job?

District E

CPN 1   We used to have a monthly get together and a meal after our journal club. That doesn't function now. We have our own domestic arrangement for informal 'wet' lunches.

CPN 2   I like *Classic FM*. I also have my dog for company.

CPN 3   It's essential to have a sense of humour. The monthly get together was also important. While the whole morning was taken up, it was a very valuable experience. It was the sharing and communicating that was helpful.

Summary

1. Develop a sense of humour.
2. Utilize stress reduction strategies: 'As soon as it turns 5 o'clock, I go off to the swimming pool'.
3. Talk to others about the pressures.

Question 6: What coping skills do new CPNs need?

District C

CPN 1   Time management, or you get torn all over the place, and being assertive.

CPN 2 Telephone skills.

CPN 3 Being able to ask for help, when you need it.

CPN 4 Regular supervision.

CPN 5 Orientation so you know what is going on.

Summary

1. Time management.
2. Clarity about the role of a CPN.
3. Being able to work independently in the community: 'It takes a lot of getting used to being on your own'.

Question 7: Why did you decide to become a CPN?

District E

CPN 1 Initially I worked as a ward sister in two hospitals. I knew I enjoyed working with people who had mental health problems. But I got increasingly frustrated by the red tape on the wards. I might identify something to do on the ward, yet other conflicting needs might have to take priority. In the community situations are more immediate, there is more face to face contact. People on the ward have things done to them. In the community it is a balanced approach with the client, one to one. Therapeutically it is more meaningful in the long run. You are not moulding people into a ward routine. The constraints we work under now have changed this.

CPN 2 I find there is more consistency for the clients. On the ward there is often conflict amongst the staff as to the clients' management. In the community you are the only person dealing with the patients. There may be conflict with other professions, but not with nurses.

CPN 3 On the wards more and more of my time was being taken away from clients. My skills as a mental health nurse were not being put to good use. I had to do a lot of organizing. I knew that I had the skills to work with clients, but on one occasion I was told that because a member of staff was off sick, there wasn't even time to talk to the clients.

Summary

Two main themes emerged from the comments here:

1. There is more freedom as a CPN.
2. You get away from the constraints and pressures of having to work on the ward.

Question 8: Do you think you are affected by problems outside work?

District D

CPN 1 Clients pick it up. It's awful when they draw your attention to it. People are not interested in your problems, they just talk about their own.

CPN 2 Family bereavement and grief work are difficult. You can't tell clients that you don't feel like talking about a specific problem like death, because you are dealing with it yourself. You could have four clients who have problems handling grief in one day.

Summary

1. Pressure at home affects your ability to function well at work.
2. Problems of working while bringing up a young family were cited.
3. Work with clients sometimes evokes personal traumas in professionals' lives.

Question 9: Do ethnic issues cause you any stress?

District A

CPN 1 Yes, all the time. It's frustrating and annoying. Blame it on the area we work in. There is not much done on behalf of a population which has a large ethnic mix.

CPN 2 You work with a black client. Maybe it should be a black CPN. I feel worried about it.

CPN 3 I was intimidated by a client who had a swimming pool. He came out with a glass of whisky. I thought, I don't belong to this class.

CPN 4 There are fears that this area is dangerous. I bring students to one of the areas that has a reputation for being intimidating. However this is only a perception by certain people who wish to tarnish it in this way.

CPN 5   It's important to emphasize looking at cultural issues. A lot of clients are misdiagnosed because the cultural component is overlooked.

CPN 6   For me, I am more aware of ethnic issues since I was mugged. I was working at the time. I had been collecting someone's money. I have had a few incidents in the past of people calling me 'chinky' but I had never been mugged before.

Summary

In several districts this was a contentious issue. Most CPNs discussed it in two main ways:

1. The effects it had on their clients: 'A client didn't understand English. We could not tell if her giggling was a sign of a deeprooted problem ... We could not find out as we could not get an interpreter quickly enough'.
2. The effects it had on them: 'I feel a sense of covert discrimination from some clients ... also from a couple of consultants'.

Question 10: Do you think stress is an important area for us to look at?

District B

CPN 1   Yes. If you don't, what often happens is people get into a defensive way of working, which doesn't do the client or CPN any good. If people are overwhelmed with clients, they manipulate clients off their caseload.

CPN 2   Not looking at stress is denying existing real stressors we are all presented with. It could lead to individuals invalidating feelings and could be self-destructive.

CPN 3   There are practical things. If people are stressed they take time off sick. They absent themselves in different ways, such as not supporting colleagues, being unhappy, staying away from work. It's a vicious circle.

CPN 4   Stress doesn't seem to be acknowledged on the wards. 'Don't cry about it.' People talk. They say, 'You chose to be a psychiatric nurse, you should expect to be hit from time to time.' It is seen as a sign of weakness to express that you are under stress.

Summary

There was widespread agreement that stress was an important issue for us to be researching. CPNs cited the following reasons as most important:

1. Stress affects your health.
2. The work of a CPN is stressful.
3. Examining stress may lead to healthy restructuring of the job.
4. Stress affects team morale and absenteeism.

Question 11: Do you have personalities prone to stress?

District B

CPN 1   Yes we wouldn't be in the job if we didn't.

CPN 2   I don't feel personally that I am very prone to stress.

CPN 3   If you don't get stressed in this job, then you are psychotic! Luckily our recruitment is of people with neurotic character structures and not people with psychotic problems.

Summary

Responses to this question were also polarized:

1. Several CPNs felt that they were emotionally stable as a group.
2. Other CPNs felt that they were a bit unbalanced themselves, but that this was an inevitable feature of the work.

Question 12: Are there any improvements you would like to make to your work?

District B

CPN 1   Yes, we would like some extra staff.

CPN 2   Maybe we could get rid of a lot of the paperwork.

CPN 3   We could look at the limitations of care. We would review how long we keep clients on for to be most cost effective.

CPN 4   Maybe we should try to get consultants to see that we can't actually do any more. We are already overloaded.

CPN 5   It might be easier if the only referral route was via the GP. We don't have an open referral system. The chosen few know about the system.

CPN 6 We need a better structure. We should think about the Patient's Charter and about purchasers defining what they want to buy from us.

CPN 7 We are a specialist service, so we should be using our skills appropriately. Maybe we should only see clients with the most serious disorders and not just anyone who has an emotional problem.

Summary

Three main themes arose here:

1. Reduce caseloads.
2. Increase the availability of back-up resources: 'A better system for getting clients back into hospital'.
3. Better working conditions.

FINDINGS FROM THE INDIVIDUAL INTERVIEWS

The individual interviews were based on 21 questions, fairly similar to those used in the group discussion. Rather than going through all the answers to each question for all the individuals surveyed, we will present a case study. The CPN in this case study was aged 42 and had been working in the community for nine years. She is a team leader in charge of six CPNs and she works in an inner city setting. She is an H Grade. One or two minor details of the interview have been altered to protect her confidentiality.

Interviewer What aspects of your job cause you most stress?
CPN Recently our management structure changed. My line manager lost her job. I was put in charge of the team without having adequate preparation and training.

   The fact is that now there are fewer beds, people are admitted, treated and discharged before they are well. They come to us. My colleagues say we don't have the resources, but legislation dictates what we must do.

   In management terms, I felt I had to produce the goods or else I would be the next one in line. I don't know what will happen to jobs in the next six months. There aren't enough resources. If we can't do it, then will it tell on us?

   Other aspects of the Community Care Act legislation can be stressful. For instance, Section 117, with the key worker being assigned. The wards often think it should

	be a CPN, but without actually telling the CPN. I found it stressful when the CPNs come to me because of this.
Interviewer	Can you describe a recent incident that has been very stressful for you?
CPN	Somebody was recently referred to us. The CPN sent them an appointment. If the patient does not attend then we assume they are okay. In this case the CPN sent three appointments but did not get a reply. The CPN then informed the referrer of this outcome. The referrer wrote back saying the CPN should have been more assertive. The CPN was hurt by this as they had tried hard. I advised the CPN to invite the referrer on a joint visit.
Interviewer	What aspects of the work of a CPN do you think your colleagues find most stressful?
CPN	The lack of resources. The sheer volume of referrals, especially now when dealing with very ill people who are difficult to discharge from our services.
Interviewer	Is working as a CPN more stressful than working on the ward?
CPN	In a way, yes. You are responsible for your caseload, for making decisions and taking flak from referrers. On the ward, you can have a stressful shift, but you can hand responsibility to someone else. Being a CPN is a 24-hour responsibility.
Interviewer	If you were having a problem at work, is there anybody that you could talk to about it?
CPN	My colleagues.
Interviewer	How would you describe the level and type of support you get at work?
CPN	My manager does not have health service experience. I don't have any clinical input. No-one therefore supervises or advises me. It is currently being looked at. I tend to discuss my own problems with my colleagues.
Interviewer	Do you think you are affected by problems outside work?
CPN	Not all the time. When I've had a crisis I think about it at home. It does not interfere though with my domestic life.
Interviewer	How do you generally cope with the stress of your job?
CPN	If I have had a particularly stressful day, I listen to music to distract myself. Alternatively I will call one of my colleagues.
Interviewer	Do you think that your coping skills are effective in controlling the stress of your job?

CPN	For myself – yes. The following day I feel okay, especially if I've talked to one of my colleagues. I find these coping methods work, so I keep on using them.
Interviewer	Do you ever use smoking or drinking or overeating as strategies to help you cope when you are under pressure?
CPN	No, none of them.
Interviewer	Does your manager cause you additional stress in your job?
CPN	My manager came from industry. He asks me to do certain things that I have not been trained for. I could ask for help, but what would he think of me if I was asking for help all the time? The manager seems to think that all I have to do is go on a business management course and then I will be properly equipped to handle all my new responsibilities.
Interviewer	What could your manager do to reduce stress at work?
CPN	If I ask for help, then he helps me. I would have preferred it if he had asked me about taking on the new responsibilities before landing them on me.
Interviewer	How well would you say you coped with problems outside of work?
CPN	I don't bring problems to work. The only time when I feel a bit stressed is if my children are unwell. If they are that ill that I can't send them to the childminder's or school, it means that I have to take some of my annual leave to cover.
Interviewer	Do you think that ethnic issues cause you any stress as a CPN?
CPN	Where clients are concerned. If I find a resource that I feel will be helpful for them. Occasionally they might reject it because they don't fit in. This I find stressful. Speaking personally as a West Indian CPN I have not experienced racism or sexism. Most of my clients are simply happy to have someone there who cares.
Interviewer	Has the stress of your job as a CPN ever made you feel that it was the wrong job for you?
CPN	No. Not after being on the wards.
Interviewer	Why did you decide to become a CPN?
CPN	When I was working on the wards, I heard about a colleague doing the CPN course. It sounded really interesting to me. I applied and got a place. I then did the

	CPN course before working in the community. I have never looked back.
Interviewer	Do you think your job is especially stressful at the moment?
CPN	Yes, lots of referrals are waiting, but all the CPNs have full caseloads. You get phone calls saying that it's urgent. We don't have the time or resources. Knowing the GPs are fundholders is worrying. If we don't respond to their requests how will they rate our services?
Interviewer	Do you feel that stress is an important issue for us to look at?
CPN	Yes it needs looking at, particularly now with the Community Care Act. If people are stressed all the time they will burn out quickly and lose enthusiasm for the job.
Interviewer	Do you feel you have a personality particularly prone to stress?
CPN	It takes a lot for me to be stressed. I suppose coming again from experience I was well prepared for it. I was the only sister in a family of six brothers. I think I had a good apprenticeship. I don't think I have a personality prone to stress.
Interviewer	Are there any improvements you have thought about making to the way you work?
CPN	I suppose doing training courses and workshops on management would help me. If I spaced out my supervision sessions with my colleagues, that might help.
Interviewer	Is there anything you feel you would like to talk about in relation to stress?
CPN	With all the organizational changes happening, it would help if CPNs could be more seriously involved and heard by the planners. Don't forget they have already been working in the community for some time now. The community base we had before was unsuitable. We told the managers this, but they didn't listen. We also suggested that the service be neighbourhood or sector based, so that CPNs could more easily get around their own patch.
Interviewer	That is all the questions I have for you. Thank you very much for participating.

Comments

Individual interviews, not surprisingly, all differed. In the above case study, clearly the CPN was affected by managerial changes within the service. She was clearly apprehensive about the new manager from outside the health service. Her concerns were largely centred around this issue. Four months after this interview was conducted she left the health service completely to return to the West Indies to take up a teaching post!

FINDINGS FROM THE DEMOGRAPHIC QUESTIONNAIRE

The previous chapters (6 and 7) have presented information on the demographic make-up of the sample. In this section we report on the responses of the CPNs to the question, 'What would you say are the three most stressful things in your job as a CPN?'. This was a question that was asked previously by West and Savage (1988) in their study of stress in health visitors.

Table 8.1: The most stressful aspects of the job as a CPN

		% of CPNs reporting the item
1	Caseload	24
2	Paperwork – administration	22
3	Management problems	18
4	Lack of resources within the community	13
5	Current changes in the NHS	13
6	Travel – traffic/parking/distance	11
7	Inadequate support	10
8	Working environment – lack of facilities	10
9	Lack of staff numbers	10
10	Time management – trying to fit it all in	10
11	Isolation of the work	9
12	Staffing problems – conflict/bickering	9
13	Number of referrals	8
14	Uncertainty over future – with job	8
15	Violent, aggressive or demanding clients	7
16	Clients in general	7
17	Problems with other disciplines	6
18	Inadequate or absent communications	6
19	Keeping notes up to date	5
20	Uncertainty over the direction of the service	4

The responses in Table 8.1 were generated by the CPNs themselves and were elicited prior to their being given the CPN Stress

Questionnaire to complete. It is interesting, therefore, to note the degree of overlap between this list and the top ten stressors from our questionnaire (see Table 7.7). Perhaps the biggest difference between the lists is in the profile of management. For instance, the third most stressful item on this list was 'Management problems' such as having 'incompetent senior management'. Item 5 – 'Current changes in the NHS' – was also a cause for concern.

No doubt closely linked to this was item 14 – 'Uncertainty over the future with the job'. It will not hurt to reiterate the point made in Chapter 7 that 52% of CPNs did not feel secure in their job. Resource issues were also paramount. Item 4 – 'Lack of resources in the community' – and item 9 – 'Lack of staff numbers' – illustrated this concern. Lack of adequate staff support also came out as an issue of concern.

A second question from the Demographic Questionnaire that we examined was, 'What helps you cope best with the pressures of your job?'. Table 8.2 presents the major responses. The issue of support was clearly critical. CPNs drew their support from a variety of sources. Support from colleagues was clearly the most frequent response, cited by 42% or 104/250 people who participated in the study. Support was also seen as coming from managers, friends and partners, in almost equal proportions.

Table 8.2: CPNs' favoured coping strategies

		% of CPNs reporting the item
1	Support from colleagues	42
2	Supervision	13
3	Keeping strict boundaries	7
4	Sport activities	7
5	Support from other disciplines	6
6	Family support	5
7	Hobbies/interests	5
8	Support from partner	5
9	Support from manager	4
10	Support from friends	4

Supervision was the second most frequently rated response. Perhaps one of the most encouraging and surprising features of the present study is that so-called maladaptive coping responses, such as smoking and drinking alcohol, are not in the top ten preferred coping strategies. Similarly relaxation training, a favoured technique amongst many psychologists, was only reported by two CPNs from the total sample of 250.

IMPLICATIONS FOR COMMUNITY PSYCHIATRIC NURSING

In this section we look at some of the practical implications arising from the Claybury CPN Stress Study. In Chapter 9 the issues of coping with stress will be addressed from the perspective of the research literature.

The Claybury CPN Stress Study has demonstrated that working in the community is more stressful than working in hospital settings. On Goldberg's General Health Questionnaire (GHQ-28), we found that 41% of CPNs scored at or above the caseness level, in comparison with 28% of ward staff. CPNs are often called on to help clients in the community manage their stress levels. Is there any element, therefore, of CPNs not practising what they preach? Do CPNs allow time for rest and relaxation? Do they pay attention to a healthy diet? Do they take regular exercise? Do they restrict their use of cigarettes and alcohol? Do they recognize their own limits?

Clearly CPNs were utilizing some coping strategies effectively to manage their stress at work. In the previous section we reported how 42% of CPNs utilized support from colleagues as a preferred coping strategy. Equally positively, some 13% of CPNs recognized the value of supervision as a positive strategy in handling stress. Part of the reason for developing our CPN Stress Questionnaire was to identify the specific occupational stressors that CPNs experienced in their work. In Chapter 7, Brown and Leary described what the ten most stressful events were for CPNs. We will now look at each of these in turn and will make some recommendations as to how the stresses might be ameliorated.

1. Not having facilities in the community that you can refer clients on to

In practical terms this may be manifested in 'stagnant' caseloads and ever lengthening waiting lists. Clearly feeding back this information to purchasers is of the utmost importance. In such circumstances CPNs also need to be aware of their own limitations and accept that they cannot go on adding clients to their caseloads ad infinitum. Acceptance of this fact can lead to reduced stress from frustration and guilt.

The need to set targets for CPN interventions is important. If long-term mental illness is the target population, then CPNs may have to admit that a proportion of their cases will remain static. The issue then becomes one of 'case mix' – what proportion of the total caseload should these clients form?

2. Knowing there are likely to be long waiting lists before clients can get access to services

This item is clearly linked to the first one, for instance, knowing that there is a nine month waiting list for assessment for psychotherapy. The CPN has to maintain contact with the client until their assessment interview comes up and even then there is no guarantee they will be accepted for psychotherapy. CPNs are not in a position to generate new services themselves. Again, communicating information to other disciplines about the limits of the CPN service and where hold-ups are occurring may defuse the build-up of stress. The support of management is also critical. This stressor reflects a failure of the community care system, rather than of individual CPNs.

3. Having to deal with suicidal clients on your own

The nature of psychiatric problems is such that suicide is always an occupational concern. Indeed, the government sees the reduction in suicide rates as being one of the main targets in its *Health of the Nation* report. Several CPNs reported this as a concern in their individual interviews.

> A client took an overdose. This stressed me as I worried whether they had taken an overdose because I had neglected them. Was I doing enough for them? The problem is you have so much to do.

Clearly, training in how to assess suicide risk and being able to discuss the issues openly is very important. Previous experience in dealing with similar situations is also a critical factor in how individual CPNs cope. As CPNs are often working in isolation in the community, it is imperative that they are able to discuss handling potentially suicidal patients, with opportunities to discuss their reactions to the incident should it occur.

4. Not having enough time for study or self-improvement

The importance of postqualification training is increasingly being recognized. Good training increases the confidence of staff and can reduce stress. Management can also help by providing relevant occupational journals for staff, funding for external training courses and allowing time for study.

5. Trying to keep up a good quality of care in your work

Increasing pressure to enlarge caseload size would seem to make it harder for CPNs to maintain the same quality of care in their work. By definition, 40 clients cannot receive as good a service as 20. Caseload monitoring would seem to be important here. An upper ceiling may need to be put on the number of clients each CPN should be seeing regularly. Attention also needs to be paid to the 'demandingness' of each client. A CPN may only have a caseload of ten but they could be the most difficult community clients in the service. A balance therefore needs to be struck between numbers and types of client, to ensure that CPNs are able to work to their optimum level.

6. Having too many interruptions when trying to work in the office

There are a number of practical ways of dealing with interruptions in the office. Firstly CPNs might set up a rota system to answer the phones at peak times. Secondly secretaries might be able to screen incoming calls. They might also be able to help minimize the disruption caused by endless streams of visitors. Partitioning of office space may be necessary to reduce the distraction of certain types of office equipment such as photocopiers or noisy dot matrix printers. Time management skills (Fontana, 1993) also extend to telephone behaviour.

7. Having to visit unsafe areas

The main difficulty here is having to visit clients who live in troublesome and dangerous housing estates. This is much more threatening to the CPN than the client themselves. Joint visits to see such clients are unfortunately costly, often impractical and difficult to arrange. Calling in to the office after such visits, assuming the CPN can find a working phone, can help keep colleagues at base briefed as to how the CPN is getting on.

8. Feeling there is not enough hospital back-up

While CPN services are still in an embryonic phase of development and as long as a lot of resources are still locked up in the hospital system, this will remain problematic. Good communication between CPNs, GPs and psychiatrists can improve the situation considerably, enabling a much quicker response to crises and sometimes obviating the need for admission. It will also help if ward staff spend some time in the community and CPNs occasionally work back on the ward. It must be recognized that ward staff on acute wards are under considerable pressure themselves.

9. Having to work with a client with a known history of violence

Containing and managing violence in hospital settings is clearly something that hospital based psychiatric nurses have become accustomed to over the years. Many ward staff have attended 'control and restraint' courses. Many options, such as having extra staff, are not available to CPNs in the community. Where there is a serious concern about a particular client, then joint visits may be the only available option. This is clearly a very important training issue.

10. Having to cope with changes in your workbase

It is sometimes stated that CPNs do not need offices as they should be working out in the community. Clearly all CPNs need an office base. It is only rarely that CPNs have full access to the range of support services, such as adequate secretarial back-up. Some CPNs are lucky to have their own desk!

CONCLUDING COMMENTS

In this chapter we started off by examining the qualitative data that emerged from group discussions with CPNs. We then looked at a case study of an individual interview with a CPN. These data have provided us with valuable insights into how CPNs perceive their role. They have helped enhance our understanding of stress and coping amongst CPNs.

We then looked at what CPNs felt were the three most stressful aspects of their job. This self-generated list of stressors overlapped closely with the items reported as being stressful from our own questionnaire.

In terms of how CPNs coped with the pressures of their work, support from colleagues was by far the most important coping strategy. This is an issue that Sue Ritter and her colleagues will address in Chapter 9.

Finally, we examined how CPNs might cope with the ten highest rated stressors from our questionnaire. Clearly, stress is a concern for CPNs. The isolated nature of their work, often in challenging urban environments with difficult patients, no doubt means that stress is probably a necessary occupational hazard. As the Director of the Hospital Advisory Service has suggested that the CPN is the single most important professional involved with care in the community, perhaps it is now time that their efforts are given the full recognition they deserve in terms of better resourcing.

Acknowledgements

We are grateful to all the CPNs who participated in the group discussions and interviews. Dr Susan Beardsell and Dr Colin Sanderson gave us helpful advice in setting up the study. Norma Matthews provided secretarial back-up.

REFERENCES

Fontana, D. (1993) *Managing Time*, BPS Publications, Leicester.
Gallagher, T. (1992) *A Q-methodological study of stress and coping mechanisms in the community psychiatric nurse*. Unpublished BSc thesis, University of East London.
Goldstein, H. (1993) The qualitative research report, in *Professional Writing for the Human Services*, (ed. L. Beebe), NASW Press, Washington.
Leary, J., Gallagher, T., Carson, J. et al. (1994) The use of Q-methodology to look at stress and coping in CPNs. *Journal of Advanced Nursing* (in press).
Silverman, D. (1993) *Interpreting Qualitative Data*, Sage, London.
Stephenson, W. (1936) A new application of correlations to averages. *British Journal of Educational Psychology*, 6, 43–57.
West, M. and Savage, Y. (1988) Stress in health visiting: qualitative accounts. *Health Visitor*, 61(9), 305–8.

CHAPTER 9

Coping with stress in mental health nursing

Susan A. Ritter, Barry Tolchard and Roisin Stewart

INTRODUCTION

'Active coping' may be defined as being in a state of readiness to undertake (difficult) tasks or to meet a challenge (Van Doornen and Van Blokland, 1992). Active coping includes an engagement with the task or challenge to achieve desired or desirable goals: so that engagement may be understood to include a sensation of performing well, as well as obtaining a tangible reward. Although the nature of the reward is likely to affect the amount of effort expended by individuals, another effect derives from any risk involved in the challenge. A low risk, high reward challenge is likely to promote a qualitatively as well as quantitatively different effort from a high risk low reward challenge.

A good deal of information about coping strategies comes from research into people's responses to chronic and fatal disease. For instance, responses of people with cardiovascular disease have been identified as defensive coping and classified as 'denial of illness' and 'repressive coping' (Warrenburg *et al.*, 1989). A fairly consistent feature of the research into stress and coping of psychiatric and mental health nurses is the incompleteness of data resulting from non-participation by respondents. It is an open question whether reluctance to take part in studies of stress is evidence of a coping style characterized by repression and denial.

Perceptions of both risk and reward may be affected by the individual's state as well as by the degree of perceived threat, so that motivation cannot simply be quantified in terms of the risk/reward ratio. The direction of influence between an individual's perceptions or attributions and their psychophysiological state cannot be assumed to be linear, one-way or stable. Tasks and other life events may have non-specific effects which challenge one or more systems, whether the cardiovascular system, immune response or neuroendocrine response. It appears that these effects are modulated by complex patterns of catecholamines, peptide hormones, corticosteroids and immunoglobulins whose levels and actions vary according to the acuity or chronicity of a given stressor (Brehm and Self, 1989).

A transactional view of stress (where behavioural, psychological and physiological responses covary) allows flexible definitions of coping at the expense of specific information with which to make decisions about optimal coping strategies. In effect, most advice to psychiatric and mental health nurses tends, like their own interventions with clients and patients, to be based on commonsense interpretations of the implications of the available literature. For example, Wright, Williams and Dill (1992) suggest that moderately difficult challenges elicit active coping where easy, extremely difficult and impossible challenges do not.

Active coping may be subdivided into three components. An 'effortful approach' suggests the engagement with the task mentioned above. Additionally, there are two kinds of avoidant coping strategies. An active strategy, while avoiding engaging with the task, is directed at avoiding an aversive outcome. A passive strategy avoids engaging with the task and may succeed also in avoiding the aversive outcome as well. It is possible that the avoidance of face-to-face contact with patients that has been observed in a number of studies of psychiatric nursing practice is a form of this avoidant coping.

A number of other studies have classified coping strategies differently. In a study of 742 adults aged over 50, Rohde *et al.* (1990) identified three coping factors associated with stress and depression: 'Cognitive self-control, 'ineffective escapism' and 'solace seeking'. Ineffective escapism exacerbated the negative impact of stress on depressed mood. Solace seeking appeared to buffer the effect of stress on depressed mood. In a study of people with chronic obstructive airways disease Lane and Hobfoll (1992) found that the disorder reduced the resources available to patients at the same time that its symptoms further restricted and frustrated them. Their anger alienated people who might otherwise have provided social support, further reducing their perceived resources.

This cycle of stress, loss, increased stress and increased loss may be evident in other groups. McCarroll *et al.* (1993) found that workers handling the bodies of people who had died in violent circumstances such as aeroplane crashes and explosions coped with their duties by using strategies such as avoidance, coping and support from their wives and husbands. They suggest that denial is a 'natural' coping mechanism and that much work remains to be done on the nature of any support given to workers under extreme stress. On the basis of their findings that female home-care workers with the elderly in New York cope with the stress they feel from their low pay and interpersonal difficulties by using strategies such as denial, identification with their clients and altruism, Bartoldus, Gillery and Sturges (1989) recommend better supervision and recognition by professional workers.

Carver, Scheier and Weintraub (1989) distinguish between problem focused coping, emotional focused coping and a third set of activities (venting emotions, behavioural and mental disengagement) which they suggest are less useful ways of coping with stress. They have developed scales to measure aspects of each type of coping. Problem focused coping includes planning and seeking instrumental social support. Emotional focused coping includes seeking emotional social support, acceptance and denial. They suggest that individuals have patterns of dispositional and situational responses to stress. Whittington and Wykes (1992) found that denial was associated with a decrease in psychological difficulties following assault by a patient.

Cranwell-Ward (1987) provides a handbook in which she has applied many of these concepts of vulnerability and coping in order that individuals can measure their own responses to stress and devise ways of modulating them. The success of her recommendations depends on the user persisting with recordings and diaries of their practice. It may be that forming a stress management group would help individuals to persevere. Another handbook (Cabinet Office, 1987) applies similar principles and could be used to supplement Cranwell-Ward's.

The scarcity of studies of psychiatric and mental health nurses which explicitly link any of these types of coping strategies for stress with the outcomes for the main tasks which nurses face means that many inferences have to be made on the basis of insufficient evidence. The main assumption of this chapter is that coping strategies modulate the nature of an individual's transaction with a stressor (Anisman and Zacharko, 1982). The definition of coping varies from study to study.

'Jobs in the NHS are by nature difficult and emotionally challenging' (Harvey, 1992). It appears that staff feel guilty when considering their own needs. They view this as a failing on their part and feel that they lose credible professional standing in the eyes of their colleagues and their superiors. However, the culture in which nursing takes place is one that seems to inhibit the development of close professional and supporting ties among nurses (Hillier, 1981), creating a greater sense of alienation and hopelessness among the 'caring' team.

CHALLENGES WHICH ELICIT COPING RESPONSES

The literature on stress among psychiatric and mental health nurses is reviewed in Chapter 3. Remaining areas of concern are shift work and work overload. As a means of providing a better service for patients there has been an increasing move towards internal rotation where nurses are expected to work both day and night shifts (Bartholomeyczik *et al.*, 1992). A mixture of day and night shifts leads to disturbed sleep patterns, disorganized diet and general levels of tiredness and fatigue. If these problems are not dealt with then the likelihood of stress and even depression amongst such workers is increased (Milne and Watkins, 1986; Glass *et al.*, 1993).

Associated with the effects of internal rotation is work overload. In one study it is proposed that 'too much work (quantitative overload) or too difficult work (qualitative overload) are two separate aspects of work overload which have been identified as related to occupational stress' (Hawkins, 1987). This is most commonly expressed by psychiatric nurses as having too little time. Internal rotation combined with other factors such as staff shortages and missing meals while at work can further increase overload.

STRATEGIES FOR MANAGEMENT OF STRESS IN PSYCHIATRIC AND MENTAL HEALTH NURSING

Active coping

The commonest intervention for reducing the physical aspects of occupational stress is to introduce some kind of stress management programme rather than to modify the working environment. Some programmes try to identify and reduce the stress rather than the stressors (Lees and Ellis, 1990; James *et al.*, 1990). Others attempt to improve the skills of the psychiatric nurses in order to reduce levels of stress (Dunne *et al.*, 1991).

Overall the main aim of these interventions is to help reduce physical reactions to stress by using a number of techniques including relaxation (MacLellan, 1990b), distraction (Burnard, 1988), exercise (Biddle and Fox, 1989), better shift patterns (Bartholomeyczik *et al.*, 1992) and help to reduce smoking (Alexander and Beck, 1990), alcohol consumption and other unhelpful lifestyle habits.

Relaxation

Although this is a very popular technique amongst clinical populations it is usually ineffective and may have the paradoxical effect of increasing anxiety in some people (Alkubasey *et al.*, 1992, Dillon, 1992). Its effects on a person's levels of stress appear to be shortlived.

Relaxation is used in occupational health settings (Skiles and Hinson, 1989; Vaughn *et al.*, 1989). Where it has been encouraged as a stress reducer within psychiatric nursing and mental health nursing the short-term results have been encouraging (Lees and Ellis, 1990). A study of a cognitive-behavioural technique of relaxation with Chinese general nurses showed a reduction in their scores on measures of stress (Tsai and Crockett, 1993). A panel design comparison of hypnosis and progressive relaxation in a single sample of American nursing students indicated that both interventions reduced psychophysiological responsivity (Forbes and Pekala, 1993). However, there are no long-term studies looking at whether beneficial effects continue.

O'Brien and van Egeren's (1991–1992) findings in college students may be relevant to the assessment of the efficacy of relaxation. They found that students with type A behaviour patterns were less likely to avoid overwork and use relaxation than students with type B behaviour patterns. This finding suggests that relaxation is better offered as part of a multifaceted intervention which addresses stress related behaviours from different angles. Johansson (1991) used such a package in an experimental study of American college based general nursing students, finding post-test that the experimental group's scores on anxiety and depression inventories were reduced. Crist *et al.* (1989) have devised a self-report measure to assess the effects of relaxation training.

Distraction

This can take many forms and its effectiveness depends on the techniques used. Within the working environment it is difficult to use such methods as a result of workload pressures mentioned earlier. However, one very useful method is to find an object in the room you are sitting in and concentrate on that object for a few minutes. If your mind wanders, gently bring yourself back to the object, noting its detail, colour, texture and shape. The aim of this technique is to distract you from your previous thoughts and to clear your mind in preparation for other things (Burnard, 1988). Most distraction methods use similar processes and can be good short-term reducers of stress. However, the long-term benefits of this have not been evaluated.

Exercise

Many occupational stress management packages have some increase in activity built into them. It is known that exercise can reduce some of the health related problems associated with stress (Biddle and Fox, 1989). Industrial companies have used this to help their workers, but mental health units are slow to catch up. The main benefits of exercise, especially in its aerobic forms, are as follows:

1. It is associated with reduced state anxiety.
2. It is associated with decreased level of mild to moderate depression.
3. It is usually associated with reductions in dysphoria.
4. It has beneficial emotional effects across all age groups and in both sexes.

(Biddle and Fox, 1989)

However, it has been shown that people who are fit and who take strenuous exercise have very different physiological responses, particularly in the immune system, from people who are not fit. Any exercise programme must be tailored for the individual, taking into account current general health status, past medical history, family history, history of injury and current position at work (Abernethy, Thayer and Taylor, 1990; Jenkins and Goldfarb, 1993).

Changing shift patterns

Three kinds of intervention are available. The first involves using a rapidly rotating shift system. Rotating from morning to evening to night shift minimizes the adjustment of circadian rhythms needed by workers. The second intervention involves allowing people to work the shifts they prefer. For example, people who like regular sleeping patterns and early rising may prefer to work morning shifts. One German study recommends that the total number of night shifts should be reduced and other stressors dealt with. These include not working alone, not carrying out special care tasks, free choice as to whether nurses do night shifts and ensuring that night workers feel secure on the site (Folkard, 1987; Hawkins, 1987; Barton and Folkard, 1991, Bartholomeyczik *et al.*, 1992).

The third intervention involves stabilizing sleeping and eating times within irregular shift patterns in order to minimize disruption to circadian rhythms (Folkard, 1987). Traditionally shiftwork in mental illness hospitals has often excluded provision for eating meals during a span of duty. A week of late shifts will be followed by a week of early shifts, or late shifts will be followed by early shifts. These sorts of duty rosters prevent stabilization of circadian rhythms and may exacerbate the effects of other stressors. The aim of the interventions listed above is to reduce the physical affects on the body of mental health workers who do internal rotation and long shifts.

Prevention of burnout

Two studies specifically address how burnout may be prevented or reduced in the mental health setting. Macinick and Macinick (1990) discuss both individual and supervisory strategies for reducing employee burnout. The individual preventive strategies they discuss are based on the principles of reality therapy (Glasser, 1978) of working within the system. These involve problem solving techniques, personal and career development and relaxation techniques. Supervisory strategies involve various organizational programmes such as in-service training and rotation of responsibilities. Other means of alleviating burnout entail morale boosting by supervisors who are advised to maintain close contact with their staff. Other suggests include 'mini seminars' on stress and burnout, orientation days and slide shows.

Milne, Burdett and Beckett (1986) carried out one of the few studies whereby a stress reduction intervention was actually implemented and evaluated. Nurses were asked to complete an inventory which on analysis yielded a breakdown of the main problem areas of individual patients and of the whole group. Patients who had similar problems were regrouped into the same ward. The rationale for this was that in the long-term, stress resulting from too many work tasks and inadequate staffing would be reduced. In addition, nurses were given training in behaviour therapy to increase their skills and therefore give them better preparation for dealing with patient problems. Milne *et al.* (1986) found that absenteeism/sickness rates on the wards which had shown most interest in the changes had decreased as opposed to the 'no change' wards. Unfortunately the methods of this study are flawed. Although measures of strain were used to differentiate strained and unstrained nurses as shown by absenteeism records, different measures were used to evaluate the interventions. Also when developing the distinguishing factors between strained and unstrained groups of nurses, there was a large difference in the response rates of the two groups.

Trygstad (1986) identified three main coping strategies in her study. These were:

1. self-talk, mental work with one's own perceptions and expectations;
2. taking an active role, doing something behaviourally;
3. talking to others.

Sullivan's (1993) findings on coping were inconclusive except to say that both problem focused and emotion focused strategies were used by nurses in his sample.

Avoidant coping

From the theoretical background it is possible to predict that some people may have certain cognitive or behavioural styles that may produce a higher risk of their becoming stressed under certain circumstances. Several studies have tried to evaluate this in the nursing field, but most have looked at broad nursing populations (Glass *et al.*, 1993; Plant *et al.*, 1992; Hipwell *et al.*, 1989) and only a few at mental health nursing (Jones *et al.*, 1987; Sullivan, 1993). None has looked specifically at the individual characteristics of the nurses, but it is possible to highlight a number of possible areas of vulnerability in which certain nurses may be affected by stress.

Smoking, alcohol and illicit drug use

Exposure to cigarette smoke and alcohol have been implicated in oxidative damage to cells, itself thought to be part of the physiology of stress and ageing, as well as a reactive process which may result in disorders such as cancer, atherosclerosis and neurodegenerative disease (Bjorneboe and Bjorneboe, 1993). Smoking and alcohol/drug use are often cited by nurses as their method of choice of coping (Lees and Ellis, 1990; Plant *et al.*, 1992). It appears that the use of smoking whilst working is still widespread in mental health settings. Forbidding smoking at work may have the effect of increasing within-work stress whilst making the working environment an otherwise healthier place. Ideally, smoking prevention programmes include cessation programmes especially for smokers, combined with education about alcohol use.

In one study, where a comparison was made between different groups of nurses, it was found that male nurses tended to drink more to alleviate certain work related stressors such as conflict with other nurses. It was also found that those men regarded as heavy drinkers (50+ units/week) were more likely to show higher levels of work related stress than light drinkers (Plant *et al.*, 1992). In the same study it was found that women mental health nurses were generally more likely to be heavy drinkers, smokers and users of illicit drugs than women in other nursing fields. However, the study did not determine whether this higher level of mood altering chemicals preceded nursing and could therefore be seen as a possible indicator for the kind of person entering the profession. Schill and Beyler (1992) suggest, for instance, that a 'self-defeating personality' is associated with less adaptive coping strategies such as drug and alcohol use which they found was also associated with denial and mental disengagement.

Schnall *et al.* (1992) define job strain as 'high psychological demands and low decision latitude'. They found that job strain alone or alcohol use alone was not associated with the stress indicator of raised systolic ambulatory blood pressure. However, men in high strain jobs who drank regularly had a raised blood pressure. Increased systolic ambulatory blood pressure was also associated with smoking. Left ventricular hypertrophy is associated with hypertension and may account for the relationship observed between stress and sudden death.

Nutrition

A lot of the hard evidence about immunoreactivity and cell oxidation comes from *in vitro* and non-human animal studies. Experimental work in human beings has yielded contradictory results which are likely to be explained by variability between the populations studied – variability whose nature remains to be elucidated. This means that advice about dietary management of stress that is based on such evidence must be treated with caution. It is reasonable and safe to advise people to eat a varied diet that includes portions of fresh fruit and vegetables. It is less reasonable and possibly not safe to advise them to use high dose lipid soluble vitamin supplements (for example, vitamin E), mineral supplements (for example, selenium) or to avoid fat. It is certainly not reasonable to take vitamins with supposed antioxidant properties while continuing to smoke or continuing to drink more than recommended amounts of alcohol or both (Dickinson, 1984; Menzel, 1992; Halliwell, 1992; Cederbaum, 1991; Sies, 1991; Anderson, 1991; Warpeha and Harris, 1993). Nevertheless, as part of the kind of diet that substitutes nutrition for, say, alcohol use, attention to vitamin and mineral rich foodstuffs has much to recommend it (Burk, 1989; Bjorneboe and Bjorneboe, 1993).

Using social support to modulate the effects of stress and strain

It has been found that the level of perceived control by mental health nurses has a direct impact on levels of stress and depression (Glass *et al*., 1993). Also the level of support given to nurses can influence levels of stress. A number of studies have looked at the efficacy of staff support groups and their influence upon reducing stress. A number of factors have been identified including improving relationships, challenge, appreciation and a sense of control through identifying needs, providing support and encouraging teamwork (Jenkins and Stevenson, 1991). The structure of such groups has been outlined in a number of studies (Burnard, 1991; Spicer, 1980; James *et al*., 1990). One method of support has been to use questionnaires to identify and so address the concerns of staff. Commonly used is the Ward Atmosphere and Environment Scales developed by Moos in 1973 which looks at the difference between the real and ideal ward atmosphere and involves making attempts to close the perceived gap between them (Moos, 1973; Milne, 1984; James *et al*., 1990; Tommasini, 1992).

It has rarely been shown what is required of a support group in order for it to be of any use. Most mental health units tend to put a group of staff into a room once a week and expect them to get on with it. But attempting to devise a form of support that can overcome the inhibiting nursing culture described above is not a straightforward task. Booth (1988) encountered many problems in trying to set up support groups for nurses. There was fear of being seen to need help, the hierarchical structure of nursing and a fear of loss of confidentiality. But they did achieve success with peer support groups.

EVALUATION OF A SOCIAL SUPPORT INTERVENTION

The rest of this chapter consists of an account of an intervention carried out in an inpatient setting designed to relieve stress by providing social support to the nursing staff. The study involved 25 psychiatric nurses, seven of whom took part in the intervention, and 18 of whom acted as controls. Pretest measures indicated high GHQ scores and high emotional exhaustion amongst the nurses in the intervention group. The follow-up after the intervention showed a decline in the GHQ scores and the depersonalization scores of the experimental group, while the control groups remained virtually the same.

Social support was stated as the most widely used coping strategy for nurses in the 1993 Claybury Stress Study discussed elsewhere in the book. The Claybury results indicated that out of a sample of 323 ward based psychiatric nurses, 88.9% stated social support as a useful coping strategy. It seemed logical to devise a form of support incorporating and aimed at helping to improve the use of this coping strategy. As a result of his research into stress and mental health nursing, Jerome Carson devised an approach called Social Support Intervention (Carson, 1993).

It was hoped that this form of support would help individuals enhance psychological functioning through the utilization and development of personal support systems. Its design combines a number of elements already present in some psychological therapies, such as the work of Wycherley (1987) on the development of psychoeducational models. It incorporates the insights of Yalom (1985) into the therapeutic benefits of belonging to a therapy group but it depends most on the work of Brugha *et al.* (1990) and Nichols and Jenkinson (1991) who highlight the importance of social support in the management of psychological distress and its importance in helping individuals deal with stress.

The Social Support Intervention consists of six three-hour sessions over a three week period. Each session looks at different aspects of social support. Session 1 looks at the actual concept of social support – why we need each other to cope. Session 2 consists of drawing graphs of life satisfaction, seeing people's peaks and troughs in life. In session 3 participants rank and rate the roles they play in their lives. In session 4 they map their support networks, focusing on who actually gives them support. In session 5 they look at social awareness and popularity. In the final session they are asked to set themselves goals, in an attempt to develop their own personal support networks. Participants finish the three weeks by giving their overall evaluation of the intervention.

Procedure

The nurses taking part in the intervention acted as an experimental group (Group Two). As an intervention of this particular type had not been implemented before, a set of controls was used to test its efficacy. A second ward (Group One) and a number of nurses from the original ward not involved in the study (Group Three) agreed to act as the control groups for the study.

To obtain the largest sample possible, an effort was made to give the questionnaires out to every nurse in the wards personally. The nurses were asked to complete the questionnaires that day. They did not have to put their names on them and confidentiality was strongly emphasized to all involved.

A follow-up to the initial study was carried out 6–8 weeks later to obtain post-test measures in order to assess the effect, if any, of the intervention.

Sample

The experimental group (Group Two) comprised seven psychiatric nurses who took part in the Intensive Social Support groups (six sessions in total). Out of the seven, six were women. Their ages ranged from 24 to 36. The controls (Groups One and Three) consisted of 11 nurses from another hospital in the same health authority, of whom five were women and six were men and seven nurses from the same ward as the experimental group (four women and three men). For ethical reasons the sample consisted only of those who wanted to take part. More than 60% of the regular nursing staff on each ward participated, but reluctance to respond to questionnaires was in line with other studies of nurses.

Measures

Each nurse involved in the study completed a demographic data sheet and five different questionnaires. The demographic data sheet was specific to the role of the psychiatric nurse and was based upon the demographic data sheet for CPNs, devised by Carson *et al.* for the 1993 Claybury Stress Study. The first questionnaire was the Coping Skills Questionnaire, the second was the Maslach Burnout Inventory (Maslach and Jackson, 1986), the third was the General Health

Questionnaire GHQ-28 (Goldberg and Williams, 1988); the fourth was the Minnesota Job Satisfaction Scale (Koelbel *et al.*, 1991) and the final measure was the Self-Attitude Questionnaire, a modified version of the Rosenberg Self-Esteem Scale (Wycherley, 1987). These questionnaires are described in Chapter 7.

All nurses involved in the study were given individual feedback on their questionnaire scores and two summary reports, one on the initial overall findings for the study and one on the findings for their own wards.

Results

The findings obtained from the three groups consisted of quantitative and qualitative results.

Demographic details

The average age of the respondents was 30.5 years. Both Groups 1 and 2 had a mean age of 28, whilst Group 3 was 35.8 years. The most common grade of nurse was E Grade (40% of the sample).

Qualitative results

The most stressful events as stated by all three groups were as follows.

1. Violent/aggressive incidents on the ward.
2. Time (too much to do, not enough time).
3. Actually working with the patients.
4. Shortages of either staff or resources.
5. Dealing with suicidal patients.

What is striking about these findings is the importance of clinical issues as principal stressors. This contrasts with the 1993 Claybury Stress Study on ward nurses (n = 323) and CPNs (n = 250) which indicated that administrative tasks and staffing problems generated a great deal of stress. In this study administration was the third least stressful event, probably indicating the degree of clinical responsibility that the three groups' staff have to carry. 'Lack of clinical support' was rated as the eighth most stressful event, from a list of 30 stressors.

Quantitative results

Preintervention

At the preintervention stage results among the three groups were similar. It was expected that high levels of stress within the three groups of nurses would be found (Bailey and Clarke, 1989). But the level of psychological and emotional stress was higher than expected. The average GHQ score for the whole sample was 8.3, a much higher score than that of the Claybury survey of ward based psychiatric nurses which was 3.4. Sixty six per cent of the sample scored over five, the threshold for psychiatric caseness.

The groups' scores indicate that at the outset of this study Groups Two and Three (both from the same ward) were experiencing a higher level of stress than Group One. Their scores are similar to those found by Cronin-Stubbs and Brophy (1984) in their study on burnout in psychiatric nurses in comparison to theatre nurses, ICU nurses and medical speciality nurses where the average GHQ score (using the GHQ-12) was 10.4. Cronin-Stubbs and Brophy attributed their findings to the greater level of interpersonal involvement and frequent incidents of conflict with patients and to the nurses' frustration and dissatisfaction with the large, highly structured organization in which they attempted to administer care.

The average Maslach scores indicated some cause for concern. All three groups were experiencing high levels of emotional exhaustion, high levels of depersonalization (except Group Three) and high levels of burnout in the area of personal accomplishment (except Group Two). These scores indicate high levels of burnout, alienation and low levels of empathy for clients. All groups scored similarly on job satisfaction, reporting satisfaction with their jobs generally. Extrinsic factors (e.g. salary, status) scored poorly, while intrinsic factors (e.g. achievement, recognition) scored more highly. These findings are in line with those of Cronin-Stubbs and Brophy (1984) and Bartoldus, Gillery and Sturges (1989). Self-attitude scores were around the mid-point of the scale, although those of both groups in the intervention ward indicated a slightly poorer self-attitude than that of Group One. All three groups scored similarly on coping skills.

Postintervention

Because the size of the sample was small and was non-randomly selected the changes are discussed in general terms. No conclusions can be drawn about whether the results are representative of the population from which the sample was drawn or about their probability. Group One's (the control group from the non-intervention ward) scores were unchanged from those at time one, except that their scores on time management had improved. Both the control (Group Three) and the experimental group (Group Two) from the intervention ward showed improved scores on most of the measures, with Group Two showing most improvement. Groups Two and Three improved in the areas of depersonalization and personal accomplishment, resulting in generally improved ratings on the Maslach Burnout Inventory. The most striking difference, however, was in the GHQ scores for the experimental group. All nurses scored at lower levels so that where, preintervention, six of them had reached caseness on the GHQ, postintervention only two nurses reached caseness.

Discussion

Evidence that intensive social support may be an effective form of stress management is seen in the experimental group's postintervention scores. The fall in their GHQ score indicates that their level of psychological distress has fallen after the intervention. The fall in their level of depersonalization from high to moderate may indicate that following the decline in their stress levels, they feel more able to empathize and relate to their patients. This may indicate that implementing self-care for nurses enables them to ensure both professional survival and a high standard of care for patients (Harvey, 1992). It looks as though effects of the intervention were reflected in the changes found in Group Three. Although it was a control group, it consisted of nurses from the same ward as the experimental group. The decline in their GHQ scores and their level of burnout in personal accomplishment is possibly a result of being directly affected by their colleagues' new outlook on their job and its difficulties. This indicates the importance of having an 'independent' control group (Group One) in order to test the effectiveness of the intervention.

The postintervention scores for Group One showed no difference from their scores at the baseline, apart from the improvement in time management. They still had high levels of burnout in emotional exhaustion, depersonalization and personal accomplishment, indicating that these nurses were still feeling emotionally drained, alienated and frustrated with a job they felt no sense of achievement in. Fortin (1992) equates stress management with time management. For these nurses at least, improved time management made no difference at all to their other measures of stress.

Drawbacks of the study

A larger sample size would have been more appropriate to test the efficacy of the intervention and a randomized control design would have been better than the design described here. It is not possible to know in what way the sample is biased – maybe only those with high stress levels participated? To overcome some of the shortcomings a further follow-up should occur at a later date, to see whether or not the differences between the three groups remain.

Implications of the study

It is interesting to speculate that if six three-hour sessions appear to effect quite large changes in a variety of measures, how much more could be achieved if the principle of social support and stress management was generally recognized and acted upon. In 1990 it was claimed that the NHS was an organization saturated with 'staff first' rhetoric but no discernible action (Newnes, 1990). In 1980 Gowler & Legge had suggested that unless the conflict between professional values and the demands of patient care was resolved health workers were likely to become 'suitable cases for treatment' (p. 237).

Fourteen years later, little or no progress has been made in introducing more active coping practices for NHS staff as well as patients. The feeling amongst the nurses involved in the Social Support Intervention was that they had been neglected for too long. One nurse observed, 'We should not be left to feel alone in the midst of all the workers ... used and abused ... but rather valued, cared for and supported'. This assertion does not need a complicated justification by means of research.

REFERENCES

Abernethy, P.J., Thayer, R. and Taylor, A.W. (1990) Acute and chronic responses of skeletal muscle to endurance and sprint exercise. *Sports Medicine*, **10**(6), 365–89.

Alexander, L.L. and Beck, K. (1990) The smoking behaviour of military nurses. *Journal of Advanced Nursing*, **15**, 843–9.

Alkubasey, T., Marks, I.M., Logsdail, S. *et al.* (1992) The role of exposure homework in phobia reduction: a controlled study. *Behaviour Therapy*, **23**, 559–621.

Anderson, R. (1991) Assessment of the roles of vitamin C, vitamin E, and beta-carotene in the modulation of oxidant stress mediated by cigarette smoke-activated phagocytes. *American Journal of Clinical Nutrition*, **53**(1) (Supplement), 358S–361S.

Anisman, H. and Zacharko, R.M. (1982) Depression: the predisposing influence of stress. *Behavioural and Brain Sciences*, **5**, 89–137.

Bailey, R. and Clarke, M. (1989) *Stress and Coping in Nursing*, Chapman & Hall, London.

Bartholomeyczik, S., Dieckhoff, T., Drerup, E. *et al.* (1992) Job satisfaction of night nurses in Germany. *International Nursing Review*, **39**(1), 27–31.

Bartoldus, E., Gillery, B. and Sturges, P.J. (1989) Job-related stress and coping among home-care workers with elderly people. *Health and Social Work*, **14**(3), 204–10.

Barton, J. and Folkard, S. (1991) The responses of day and night nurses to their work schedules. *Journal of Occupational Psychology*, **64**(3), 207–18.

Biddle, S.J.H. and Fox, K.R. (1989) Exercise and health psychology. *British Journal of Medical Psychology*, **62**, 205–16.

Bjorneboe, A. and Bjorneboe, G. (1993) Antioxidant status and alcohol related diseases. *Alcohol and Alcoholism*, **28**(1), 111–16.

Booth, K. (1988) Stress and nurses. Nursing, 3(28), 1017–20.

Brehm, J. and Self, E. (1989) The intensity of motivation. Annual Review of Psychology, 40, 109–31.

Brugha, T., Bebbington, P., Sturt, E. et al. (1990) The relation between life events and social support networks in a clinically depressed cohort. Social Psychiatry and Psychiatric Epidemiology, 25(6), 308–13.

Burk, R.F. (1989) Recent developments in trace element metabolism and function: newer roles of selenium in nutrition. Journal of Nutrition, 119(7), 1051–4.

Burnard, P. (1988) Stress and relaxation in health visiting. Health Visitor Journal, 61(9), 272.

Burnard, P. (1991) Peer support groups. Journal of District Nursing, 9(8), 19–20.

Cabinet Office (1987) Understanding Stress, HMSO, London.

Carson, J. (1993) Manual for Social Support Group Therapy version 3.1, unpublished manuscript, Institute of Psychiatry, London.

Carson, J., Bartlett, H., Leary, J., Gallagher, T. and Senapati-Sharma, M. (1993) Stress and the community psychiatric nurse. Nursing Times, 89(3), 38–40.

Carver, C.S., Scheier, M.F. and Weintraub, J.K. (1989) Assessing coping strategies: a theoretically-based approach. Journal of Personal and Social Psychology, 56(2), 267–83.

Cederbaum, A.I. (1991) Microsomal generation of reactive oxygen species and their possible role in alcohol hepatotoxicity. Alcohol and Alcoholism, Supplement 1, 291–6.

Cranwell-Ward, J. (1987) Thriving on Stress, Routledge, London.

Crist, D.A., Rickard, H.C., Prentice-Dunn, S. and Barker, H.R. (1989) The Relaxation Inventory: self-report scales of relaxation training effects. Journal of Personality Assessment, 53(4), 716–26.

Cronin-Stubbs, D. and Brophy, E. (1984) Burnout: can social support save the psychiatric nurse? Journal of Psychosocial Nursing and Mental Health Services, 25(8), 13.

Dickinson, D. (1984) How to Fortify your Immune System, Arlington Books, London.

Dillon, K.M. (1992) Popping sealed-air capsules to reduce stress. Psychological Reports, 71(1), 243–6.

Dunne, E.A., Melinn, A., Hemphreys, T. and Quayle, E. (1991) The impact of a training course in behavioural therapy on psychiatric nurses. Irish Journal of Psychological Medicine, 8, 40–2.

Folkard, S. (1987) Circadian rhythms and hours of work, in Psychology at Work, (ed. P. Warr), Penguin, Harmondsworth.

Forbes, E.J. and Pekala, R.J. (1993) Psychophysiological effects of several stress management techniques. Psychological Reports, 72(1), 19–27.

Fortin, P.B. (1992) Routes to modify the impact of stress. Canadian Nurse, 88(8), 37–9.

Glass, D.C., McKnight, J.D. and Valdimarsdottir, H. (1993) Depression, burnout and perceptions of control in hospital nurses. Journal of Consulting and Clinical Psychology, 61(1), 147–55.

Glasser, W. (1978) Reality Therapy: A New Approach To Psychiatry, New York, Harper and Row.

Goldberg, D. and Williams, P. (1988) A User's Guide to the General Health Questionnaire, NFER-Nelson, Windsor.

Gowler, D. and Legge, K. (1980) Evaluative practices as stressors in occupational settings, in Current Concerns in Occupational Stress, (eds C.L. Cooper and R. Payne), John Wiley and Sons, Chichester.

Halliwell, B. (1992) Reactive oxygen species and the central nervous system. *Journal of Neurochemistry*, **59**(5), 1609–23.

Harvey, P. (1992) Staff support groups: are they necessary? *British Journal of Nursing*, **1**(5), 256–8.

Hawkins, L. (1987) An ergonomic approach to stress. *International Journal of Nursing Studies*, **24**, 307–18.

Hillier, S. (1981) Stresses, strains and smoking. *Nursing Mirror*, **152**(7), 25–30.

Hipwell, A., Tyler, P. and Wilson, C. (1989) Sources of stress and dissatisfaction among nurses in four hospital environments. *British Journal of Medical Psychology*, **62**, 70–1.

James, I., Milne, D.L. and Firth, H. (1990) A systematic comparison of feedback and staff discussion in changing the ward atmosphere. *Journal of Advanced Nursing*, **15** 329–36.

Jenkins, E. and Stevenson, I. (1991) A strategy for managing change: development of staff support groups. *Professional Nurse*, **6**(10), 579–81.

Jenkins, R.R. and Goldfarb, A. (1993) Introduction: oxidant stress, aging and exercise. *Medicine and Science in Sports and Exercise*, **25**(2), 210–12.

Johansson, N. (1991) Effectiveness of a stress management programme in reducing anxiety and depression in nursing students. *Journal of American College Health*, **40**(3), 125–9.

Jones, J., Janman, K., Payne, R. and Rick, J. (1987) Some determinants of stress in psychiatric nurses. *International Journal of Nursing Studies*, **24**, 129–44.

Koelbel, P., Fuller, F. and Misener, T. (1991) Job satisfaction of nurse practitioners: an analysis using Herzberg's theory. *Nurse Practitioner*, **16**(4), 43–6.

Lane, C. and Hobfoll, S.E. (1992) How loss affects anger and alienates potential supporters. *Journal of Consulting and Clinical Psychology*, **60**(6), 935–42.

Lees, S. and Ellis, N. (1990) The design of a stress-management programme for nursing personnel. *Journal of Advanced Nursing*, **15**(8), 946–61.

Macinick, C.G. and Macinick, J.W. (1990) Strategies for burnout prevention in the mental health setting. *International Nursing Review*, **37** 246–9.

MacLellan, M. (1990a) Burnout in district nurses. *Journal of District Nursing*, February, 14–18.

MacLellan, M. (1990b) Cooling burnout. *Journal of District Nursing*, April, 13–14.

Maslach, C. and Jackson, S. (1986) *Maslach Burnout Inventory*, Consulting Psychologists Press, California.

McCarroll, J.E., Ursano, R.J., Wright, K.M. and Fullerton, C.S. (1993) Handling bodies after violent death: strategies for coping. *American Journal of Orthopsychiatry*, **63**(2), 209–14.

Menzel, D.B. (1992) Antioxidant vitamins and prevention of lung disease. *Annals of the New York Academy of Sciences*, **669** 141–55.

Milne, D. (1984) Skill evaluations of nurse training in behaviour therapy. *Behavioural Psychotherapy*, **12** 142–50.

Milne, D., Burdett, C. and Beckett, J. (1986) Assessing and reducing the stress and strain of psychiatric nursing. *Nursing Times*, **82**(7), 59–62.

Milne, D. and Watkins, F. (1986) An evaluation of the effects of shift rotation on nurses' stress, coping and strain. *International Journal of Nursing Studies*, **23**(2), 139–46.

Moos, R. (1973) Conceptualizations of human environments. *American Psychologist*, **28**, 652–65.

Newnes, C. (1990) Caring for carers' needs. *Nursing*, **4**(16), 33–4.

Nichols, K. and Jenkinson, J. (1991) *Leading a Support Group*, Chapman & Hall, London.

O'Brien, W.H. and van Egeren, L. (1991–1992) Perceived susceptibility to heart disease and preventive health behaviour among Type A and type B individuals. *Behavioural Medicine*, **17**(4), 159–65.

Plant, M.L., Plant, M.A. and Foster, J. (1992) Stress, alcohol, tobacco and illicit drug use amongst nurses: a Scottish study. *Journal of Advanced Nursing*, **17**, 1057–67.

Rohde, P., Lewinsohn, P.M., Tilson, M. and Seeley, J.R. (1990) Dimensionality of coping and its relation to depression. *Journal of Personality and Social Psychology*, **58**(3), 499–511.

Schill, T. and Beyler, J. (1992) Self-defeating personality and strategies for coping with stress. *Psychological Reports*, **71**(1), 67–70.

Schnall, P.L., Schwartz, J.E., Landsbergis, P.A., Warren, K. and Pickering, T.G. (1992) Relation between job strain, alcohol and ambulatory blood pressure. *Hypertension*, **19**(5), 488–94.

Sies, H. (1991) Oxidative stress: from basic research to clinical application. *American Journal of Medicine*, **91**(3C), 31S–38S.

Skiles, L. and Hinson, B. (1989) Occupational burnout among correctional health workers. *American Association of Occupational Health Nurses Journal*, **37**(9), 374–8.

Spicer, F. (1980) A support group for health visitors. *Health Visitor*, **53** 377–9.

Sullivan, P.J. (1993) Occupational stress in psychiatric nursing. *Journal of Advanced Nursing*, **18**(4), 591–601.

Tommasini, R. (1992) The impact of a staff support group on the work environment of a specialty unit. *Archives of Psychiatric Nursing*, **6**(1), 40–7.

Tsai, S.L. and Crockett, M.S. (1993) Effects of relaxation training combining imagery and meditation on the stress level of Chinese nurses working in modern hospitals in Taiwan. *Nursing*, **14**(1), 51–66.

Trygstad, L.N. (1986) Stress and coping in psychiatric nursing. *Journal of Psychosocial Nursing*, **24**(10), 23–7.

Van Doornen, L. and van Blokland, R. (1992) The relationship between cardiovascular and catecholamine reactions to laboratory and real life stress. *Psychophysiology*, **29**(2), 173–81.

Vaughn, M., Cheatwood, S., Sirles, A.T. and Brown, K.C. (1989) The effect of progressive muscle relaxation among clerical workers. *American Association of Occupational Health Nurses Journal*, **37**(8), 302–6.

Warpeha, A. and Harris, J. (1993) Combining traditional and nontraditional approaches to nutrition counselling. *Journal of the American Dietetic Association*, **93**(7), 797–800.

Warrenburg, S., Levine, J., Schwartz, G.E. *et al.* (1989) Defensive coping and blood pressure reactivity in medical patients. *Journal of Behavioural Medicine*, **12**(5), 407–24.

Whittington, R. and Wykes, T. (1992) Staff strain and social support in psychiatric hospitals following assault by a patient. *Journal of Advanced Nursing*, **17**, 480–6.

Wright, R., Williams, B. and Dill, J. (1992) Interactive effects of difficulty and instrumentality of avoidant behaviour on cardiovascular reactivity. *Psychophysiology*, **29**(6), 677–86.

Wycherley, R. (1987) *The Living Skills Pack*, South East Thames RHA, Bexhill.

Yalom, D. (1985) *The Theory and Practice of Group Psychotherapy*, Basic Books, New York.

CHAPTER 10

Future directions in community psychiatric nursing research

Kevin Gournay

INTRODUCTION

Although this chapter concerns an area of mental health nursing research which will certainly grow in the next few years, this is not to say that there are not considerable problems and changes to be confronted. Therefore, although the tone and conclusion of this chapter is hopefully positive, no apologies are offered for pointing out areas of threat, concern and conflict.

In order to examine the future, one needs to look at several contextual matters and in particular, to examine changes in the contemporary nature of mental health care and its delivery.

KEY CHANGES IN THE CONTEXT OF MENTAL HEALTH CARE AND ITS DELIVERY

It would not be an exaggeration to say that the changes in mental health care and its delivery in the last decade have been revolutionary and the topics discussed below represent but a selection of these changes. Psychiatric historians will in future note that these changes seemed to happen very quickly but the origin of these events can probably be traced back to shortly after the Second World War. Indeed, as Stein (1991) points out, the population in state mental hospitals in the USA began to drop in 1955 and between 1965 and 1975 the numbers of patients in mental hospitals in the United States declined from 550 000 to 120 000. This rapid process of deinstitutionalization took place principally at the instigation of President Kennedy's initiatives in 1963 with the Community Mental Health Centres Act and also in a time when more money was apparently being given to mental health services. In the United Kingdom, similar processes occurred but, as usual, slightly behind those of the United States. The beginning of the community care movement of the 1960s and 1970s was a time when resources were never seen as a major problem and many of the debates concerned the nature of mental illness. To discuss the changes which have occurred, it is necessary to consider first of all the context of mental health care in modern times and secondly, the contemporary changes in delivery.

THE CONTEXT OF MENTAL HEALTH CARE

Market economics in the provision of mental health services

The reforms of the National Health Service have lead to widespread changes and the concept of letting the market decide has been of utmost importance in contemporary mental health care. This concept has led to demands for services by GPs and the general public which do not necessarily reflect the needs of the population. In particular, it could be argued that the groups with the greatest voice will attract the services of mental health professionals. In this regard, people with the less serious mental health problems, such as minor depression and general anxiety, which may affect up to one quarter of the population, will put pressure on GPs. They, in turn, will seek counselling services for these populations rather than seeking the services of mental health professionals for those people with serious and enduring mental health problems.

Community psychiatric nursing has already been affected by this trend (White, 1993). As Gournay and Brooking (1992) have shown, CPNs working with people with less serious mental health problems do so with little impact and at considerable cost. However, for the business manager of an NHS mental health trust, what is more attractive – ten sessions of anxiety management for someone suffering the trials and tribulations of a dysfunctional marriage and/or a stressful work environment or an open-ended commitment on the part of a service to look after an individual with schizophrenia who exhibits bizarre behaviour which is at times grossly antisocial and with whom it is extremely difficult to gain any sort of rapport? Certainly from the business manager's point of view, it is much easier to factor into a business plan a number of units of anxiety management training or counselling as compared with, in effect, providing an open cheque for the treatment of someone with a serious and enduring mental health problem.

The Department of Health have, rather belatedly, recognized the problem of letting the market decide in an unfettered way. In the ten-point plan for developing successful and safe community care, announced by Virginia Bottomley in August 1993, at least four of the points are specifically aimed at redressing the balance and assisting people with serious and enduring mental health problems. First there is an emphasis on the development of better information systems, including special supervision registers of patients who may be at most risk and need most support. Second, there is an ongoing review by the Clinical Standards Advisory Group of standards of care for people with schizophrenia both in the hospital and in the community (on which the author serves). Third, the plan emphasizes that health authorities and GP fundholder purchasing plans should cover the essential needs for mental health services. Fourth, there is better training for key workers in their duties in the care programme approach and the advice that the new code of practice and guidance should take account of lessons learned from the cases that have gone wrong.

Despite the safeguards announced above, it seems clear that some trusts within the newly configured health services will give poorer services to people with serious mental health problems. This is partly because the market has 'decided' and these trusts have run into financial difficulties. There have already been several cases where large numbers of community psychiatric nurses have been made redundant, not because they were not needed but because of the financial difficulties of the trust which employed them and the need to shed staff.

Changes in funding of care and treatment

Community care in the 1990s has brought with it a new method of funding of the care and treatment of the long-term mentally ill and, after many years of lobbying by various professional and user organizations, funding for long-term community care has now moved away from health authorities or commissioning agencies to social services departments. For community psychiatric nurses this represents a considerable threat for the future, as social services departments may well wish to employ as key workers or case managers people without a mental health professional training. Rather, these departments may opt to employ people with a social work background or, as has been the case with those working with people with mental handicaps, no professional background at all. It may well be that the situation as prevails in many parts of the USA, where there are very few nurses employed as case managers, will in the near future be replicated on this side of the Atlantic. Certainly one argument for employing people other than community psychiatric nurses and other mental health professionals is a financial one. At the very least, one has to assume that the clinical grading system of the 1980s, which assumed large numbers of people employed in H or I Grades, will wither in the wake of more 'market led' service planning.

Changing models of mental health problems

Twenty years ago, the nature of mental illness was the cause for much debate and certainly until the very recent past, many mental health nursing courses, and community psychiatric nursing courses in particular, had a large content which concerned social models of the causation of mental illness. The revolution of molecular genetics of the late 1980s and the vast amount of research carried out by biochemists (which have shown a range of chemical abnormalities in schizophrenia) and the research of radiologists (which has shown neuroanatomical abnormalities) have probably put social causes of major mental health problems into their proper context. Certainly, we now recognize that social factors are important but in the maintenance of mental health problems and relapse rather than in causation (for a review of this area, see Gournay, 1993).

Changes in delivery

As indicated above, White's (1993) study shows a diversity in the delivery of community psychiatric nursing services. However, crises in mental health care will lead to a much more focused delivery of service. In the first instance there will probably be, as mentioned (without apology) in several places in this chapter, an increased focus on serious mental health problems. As a consequence of this, the two key changes in delivery will be firstly, the increased use of case management and secondly, the possible increased role in drug prescribing for CPNs. With regard to case management, this is obviously an area which cannot be tackled in a chapter such as this but it is worth mentioning some of the key concepts. Firstly, the key objectives of case management are:

1. to meet individual care needs through the most effective use of resources;
2. to restore and maintain independence by enabling people to live in the community whenever possible;
3. to minimize and prevent the negative effects of disability, illness or mental distress in people of all ages;
4. to achieve equal opportunities for all;
5. to promote individual choices of determination and build on existing strengths and care resources;
6. to promote partnerships between users, carers and service providers in all sectors.

These laudable aims are being reached by a number of stages and while these are described differently in various documents, perhaps the best contemporary description is that of Thornicroft (1994). In this article, Thornicroft lists the stages of care management and assessment as:

1. publishing information;
2. determining the level of assessment;
3. assessing need;
4. care planning;
5. implementing the care plan;
6. monitoring;
7. reviewing.

There seems little doubt that not only does case management represent a major challenge for mental health nursing in the future, but it may well become synonymous with it.

With regard to prescribing functions, it has long been accepted that in many cases, community psychiatric nurses do, in effect, alter prescriptions of psychotropic medication. In particular, CPNs are trusted by psychiatrists to give definitive views on medication and psychiatrists very often follow CPNs advice. Nevertheless, there is absolutely no reason to become complacent. The study by Bennett (1991) reveals that the community psychiatric nurses' knowledge of psychotropic medication and side effects does, in many cases, leave much to be desired and there is obviously a need for CPNs to be much more informed about the nature of medications and possible side effects. At the present time this is of paramount importance as there are now new generations of neuroleptic agents, all with their own distinct action and adverse reactions. Having made the point that CPNs have to make up some ground, there is nevertheless a very strong argument for training some CPNs to have a legal prescribing function and, given the very large numbers of people with serious mental health problems who will be in receipt of community care and therefore no longer captive as compliant hospital patients, this innovation is entirely logical.

SHORTCOMINGS OF PREVIOUS RESEARCH IN COMMUNITY PSYCHIATRIC NURSING

Although it would be easy to criticize community psychiatric nursing research over the last few years and, indeed, some of these criticisms are referred to below, it should be said from the outset that this area of research is new and therefore, as with any discipline, there are certain to be problems in evolving an identity for this area. Indeed, these problems of evolution may subsequently prove to be the basis of sound knowledge because of what has been learned in the process of working through particular difficulties.

When one considers the importance of community psychiatric nursing, the scope of the work carried out by CPNs (White, 1993) and their growing numbers, the levels of past research funding have been very low. Indeed, of the largest research grants given for topics in community psychiatric nursing, two of these have been awarded to psychiatrists; to Eugene Paykel for the Springfield trial (Paykel and Griffith, 1983) and to Isaac Marks for his study of psychiatric nurse therapists working in the community (Marks, 1985). Only one randomized controlled trial with any substantial funding (from the Department of Health) has been carried out by mental health nurses (Gournay and Brooking, 1992, 1994) while several important pieces of work have been carried out with relatively small research funds. Of these, the studies of Charlie Brooker, looking at skills for CPNs working with seriously mentally ill people (Brooker *et al.*, 1992), and the survey research of Ted White into community psychiatric nursing (White, 1993) are good examples. Jean Faugier's work on human immunodeficiency viruses (HIV) disease and drug misuse (Faugier, 1993) was funded by the Department of Health and arguably, although this work has many implications for community psychiatric nursing practice, the funds were primarily awarded for the topic of HIV rather than for nursing per se.

Further perusal of the community psychiatric nursing research literature demonstrates that most of the other work carried out has been funded with very small sums. Often the nurse researchers have given time very generously, frequently because they have been in pursuit of completing research dissertations for a higher degree. Indeed, the pursuit of a Masters degree or a PhD has, until the present time, been virtually the only training in research that community psychiatric nursing researchers – or for that matter, any mental health nursing researchers – have had. There have been a few exceptions; for example, people pursuing PhDs via Department of Health fellowships. However, after completion of a PhD there have not until the present time been any opportunities by way of postdoctoral research fellowships. As the number of researchers with doctorates grows and their experience lengthens, there should be more opportunities for postdoctoral training.

In general, the embryonic nature of the field has been reflected in deficiencies in research methodology. In particular, there has been a shortage of properly controlled experiments and very little in the way of randomized controlled trials. Past research has often been characterized by poorly controlled methods with small numbers of subjects and crude or inappropriate statistical analysis.

In the author's view, one of the biggest problems has been an encumbrance of mental health nursing research in general by the millstone of nursing models. An anecdote may serve to illustrate the point. During a visit by a member of the Joint Board of Clinical Nursing Studies (the body which preceded the English National Board) to the behaviour nurse therapy programme at the Maudsley Hospital, the nurse therapist trainees were describing their work. They explained how clients were referred to them by general practitioners and consultant psychiatrists for specialized programmes of behavioural treatment. The trainees described how assessment took place covering the client's main current problems, obtaining a picture of history and background, negotiating treatment targets with the client which were specific to the presenting problem behaviours and also reflecting general life adaptation, gathering objective data on symptom and social function levels, formulating a plan of treatment, implementing that treatment; carrying out further evaluations using multiple reliable measures of change; concluding the treatment intervention and following up the client using the same multiple and reliable measures used throughout assessment; treatment follow-up; writing letters and case summaries and communicating information on the client's progress verbally. After further detailed case examples and a description by the trainee nurse therapists of the theoretical underpinnings of this approach, the representative of the Joint Board of Clinical Nursing Studies asked 'What about the nursing process?!'.

This incident is indicative of how mental health nursing has struggled to assume an identity by using models which have been developed for general nursing. In reality, mental health nursing is but one aspect of a total process of care and treatment on conditions which have many particular aspects of both causation and manifestation. It could be argued that contemporary psychology, psychiatry and sociology provide us with enough underlying theory to understand and enquire into the nature and treatment of mental health problems. Very often the models of nursing are based on anachronistic concepts which have been long replaced by more scientifically determined theories. For example, the adaptation model of Roy (Roy, 1976, 1981) utilizes adaptation models which take no account of contemporary theories of self-efficacy, personal control and attribution theory (see, for example, Sarafino, 1990). Alternatively, nursing theorists in mental health attempt (rather badly) to create models which are independent of any prevailing psychiatric or psychological theory. For example, Orem's Self-care model (Orem, 1985) lists a number of aspects of self-care, limitations of self-care and helping methods in the context of a 'nursing system'. In the mental health nursing arena, the teaching of models such as this can only serve to confuse the student and, frankly, the espousal of the overly simplistic principles contained therein often leads to nurses being viewed as quaint but simple creatures! Obviously, the way forward is for mental health nurses to abandon these millstones and use the outcome of the longstanding research efforts of psychiatrists, psychologists and sociologists as the basis for future research and to join with them in future research endeavours.

FUTURE RESEARCH TOPICS IN COMMUNITY PSYCHIATRIC NURSING

As Julia Brooking pointed out in the introduction to her edited text *Psychiatric Nursing Research* (Brooking, 1986) there had not, until publication of this work, been any other book of its type. She made the point that the development of psychiatric nursing research lagged behind nursing research generally and that there was a lack of adequate educational opportunities available for psychiatric nurses with, at that time, only three degree programmes offered in universities or polytechnics which included registration in psychiatric nursing. Brooking made the observation that degree level study was a prerequisite for the development of research skills and added that the contributors to her text had mostly obtained degrees in other disciplines.

Reference to the two excellent texts edited respectively by Brooker (1990) and Brooker and White (1993) shows how community psychiatric nursing research has developed. While much of the research presented in these two books is of high quality and reflects the wide spectrum of activity of community psychiatric nurses, there is, at the present time, no obvious indication of which future topics will be researched. It seems vital that future research topics should reflect service developments and the results of research should have obvious consequences for practice and organization. There is no longer any room for the sort of descriptive research which leaves the reader with a 'so what?' feeling and certainly there is no place for research which aims to satisfy one or other of the anachronistic nursing models previously described. Set out below are five suggested topics for future research. There is no pretence that these are definitive in the sense of providing a comprehensive agenda. Rather, what follows are some suggestions which, it is hoped, will lead to thought and debate among community psychiatric nursing researchers. This, in turn, may lead to the formulation of research plans which should go some way towards meeting the considerable challenges of the contemporary scene.

Controlled evaluation of interventions

As White's 1990 survey of community psychiatric nursing in the UK (White, 1993) describes, community psychiatric nurses use a whole range of interventions. White reported that family therapy was the most popular approach, followed by behaviour therapy, counselling, cognitive therapy, behavioural family therapy and 14 minority approaches. Given the relatively small number of community psychiatric nurses in the UK, this is truly a bewildering array of specialist modalities. When one considers the obvious split between interventions with people with serious and enduring mental illness and those with the more minor problems of anxiety, depression and relationship difficulties, it becomes clear that there is a need to ensure that the interventions used are effective for the populations that are targeted. Gournay and Brooking (1994) show that even when one is able to evaluate the effectiveness of an intervention within the context of a randomized controlled trial, other factors may confound this evaluation. In particular, with depression and anxiety and other non-psychotic problems, there is a considerable rate of 'spontaneous remission' in up to 70% of clients seen. There is therefore a considerable need to assess the interventions used by CPNs by proper controlled enquiry.

Having said that, CPNs must also draw from already established knowledge and use research findings from other areas of professional practice. For example, it has long been established that relaxation training is an ineffective intervention in agoraphobia (Marks, 1987), that individual and group psychotherapy using an insight oriented approach is ineffective in many cases of depression and anxiety, that family therapy is unlikely to be effective in obsessive compulsive disorder if used on its own, etc, etc. Nevertheless, all of these approaches are commonly used by community psychiatric nurses and perhaps the point needs to be made that educational preparation in both the pre- and postregistration contexts for mental health nurses has never, until the present time, included sufficient detail on these and other similar research findings.

The obvious target for evaluation research is, of course, in the area of serious and enduring mental health problems. The principal areas of contemporary interest are the various cognitive behavioural interventions for positive and negative symptoms of schizophrenia, behavioural family interventions in schizophrenia and cognitive interventions in major affective disorder. It must be emphasized that there is already a considerable amount of research activity in these areas, carried out at the moment by psychiatrists and psychologists. Community psychiatric nursing researchers need to consider very seriously whether they should carry out research in isolation or whether their research endeavours should be set in the context of multidisciplinary research consortia. This of course highlights the question of whether community psychiatric nursing needs its own identity. If community psychiatric nursing researchers do pursue research within a single discipline approach, there is the danger that research may be unnecessarily replicated. On the other hand combining with researchers of other disciplines may at least strengthen the research effort and nursing may add an invaluable dimension to an already established multidisciplinary approach.

Controlled evaluation of training programmes for community psychiatric nurses

Training programmes for community psychiatric nurses have only really developed over the last two decades and there have been several changes in the curricula for the year-long ENB courses. For many reasons these courses have not been properly evaluated and there is really no evidence to hand as to whether community psychiatric nurses who have completed such courses are any more clinically effective than nurses who have not attended these courses. Gournay and Brooking (1994), with an admittedly small sample, could find no difference in outcome between a group of CPNs trained on the traditional ENB courses in community psychiatric nursing compared with CPNs without such training. Furthermore, a video analysis of the work of these two groups did not find any significant difference between the two groups. It must be said, however, that the study also showed that the approach used by both groups (i.e. client centered counselling) was ineffective. Furthermore, the research also found that those nurses who had not attended the ENB training course had had significant other training. For example, some of the CPNs in the study had trained as marriage guidance counsellors, while others had invested a considerable amount of their own money gaining additional training in various psychotherapeutic approaches.

In the last two or three years there have been some very welcome developments in training evaluations. Of individual efforts, the work of Charlie Brooker in skills acquisition with serious mental illness has been the forerunner (Brooker *et al.*, 1992). The CPNs in his study were taught to deliver various psychoeducational interventions. These included an evaluation of the needs of each family member, health education for all family members, family stress management programmes and goal setting aimed at increasing the social and personal functioning of both the client and each relative. One of the most encouraging findings of this study was that the cost of running the course was approximately £600 per student (at 1990 prices). This sum, set against the possible savings to the health care system by a reduction in relapse and therefore prevention of further and more expensive episodes of care, should be an encouragement for further investment in this sort of training. Indeed, community psychiatric nursing is currently benefiting from a very generous donation by the Sir Jules Thorn Trust to pilot the development of training programmes for mental health nurses in case management. The Thorn Programme is much more than a training in general case management skills. The pilot programme running in Manchester and London teaches skills in the range of family interventions highlighted by Brooker and also a range of psychosocial interventions aimed at reducing the impact of both positive and negative symptoms of schizophrenia (for an excellent account of these interventions, see Birchwood and Tarrier, 1992). Eventually it is hoped that the Thorn Programme will be generally available and it may well be that this form of case management training will be the single most important method of educational preparation for community psychiatric nurses.

A more in-depth training for mental health professionals, including community psychiatric nurses, has been developed by the author at Middlesex University and in this programme, experienced mental health professionals are able to undertake a two year part-time Master's degree which aims to give course graduates a range of intervention skills in serious mental health problems and also a basic training in research. The course recognized that skills in evaluation will become increasingly important for mental health nurses and the research methods component of the course aims to provide graduates with the skills and knowledge to carry out a range of quantitative and qualitative research methods. It is likely that more Master's programmes of this sort will proliferate, particularly as the demand for Master's level education will increase as graduates from the various university based nursing degree programmes begin to aspire to further knowledge and training.

Evaluation of the role of consumers in treatment

The idea that consumers of service – and sufferers of chronic mental illness at that – could be trained as case managers is revolutionary. However, as long ago as 1986 the Colorado Division of Mental Health began a pilot programme to train and employ individuals with chronic mental illness to provide case management services to other mental health consumers (Sherman and Porter, 1991). This project was carefully evaluated and two years after the project was completed, 15 of the 17 original course completers were still employed in roles best defined as that of case manager aide. One apparent benefit of training was that the whole cohort only required a total of two bed days of psychiatric hospitalization between them in the two years following training. This programme has been extended to various parts of the United States. Any possible disadvantages are more than outweighed by the benefits of such a system. Sherman and Porter point out that consumer case managers may achieve a better rapport with other consumers, may gain their co-operation with treatment programmes more readily and may help produce positive attitudes in other professionals. Furthermore, consumer case managers may help to reduce stigma and, as indicated above, the training and job experience provided may enhance the consumer case managers' own mental health states.

However, despite the recent recognition of the importance of involving users in mental health care, innovations such as this are very rare in the United Kingdom. Therefore one possible future research topic in community psychiatric nursing could be the evaluation of the role of consumers in treatment within British case management services. Community mental health nurses are uniquely placed to provide the training and supervision of such workers. Until programmes involving users in services are placed on equivalent footings to those found in many parts of the United States, it must be said that as matters stand at the present, the user presence in service provision is but token.

Research in treatment failure
(including treatment compliance and motivation)

It has been pointed out (Gournay, 1991; Gournay and Brooking, 1993) that one of the most neglected areas of outcome research in both psychiatric nursing interventions and in psychiatry generally is the issue of failure. Failure has been defined (Foa and Emmelkamp, 1983) in terms of four subgroupings. These are:

1. individuals who do not accept or refuse treatment;
2. individuals who commence treatment but drop out before an adequate trial of treatment has been completed;
3. individuals who do not respond to treatment;
4. individuals who respond to treatment but who subsequently relapse.

As the author has previously pointed out (Gournay, 1991), studies of outcome generally only follow people who complete an adequate trial of intervention but do not follow up those who drop out along the way. With particular regard to major mental health problems, this lack of compliance is a considerable issue. In community psychiatric nursing generally, it would be interesting to examine what factors correlate with poor compliance and whether there is anything that the CPN can do to increase compliance. It is of course recognized that one needs to take certain steps, such as providing information, seeing clients in their own homes, involving the family, etc. so as to engage them in treatment but surely, what is needed is much more systematic data collection and evaluation of this process.

A corollary of this of course is the client's own internal motivation process (or processes) and in this regard, clients who do not co-operate in treatment are very often written off because of 'poor motivation'. In the major mental illnesses particularly, poor motivation may indeed be part of the problem and as Birchwood and Tarrier (1992) have shown, there are now a range of cognitive behavioural procedures which may be used in helping clients deal more effectively with their symptoms. It is thus important that motivation itself is targeted as one of the problem areas. Surely, therefore, community psychiatric nurses, who will increasingly work with this population of seriously ill clients, will have a contribution to make in this research area.

Economic evaluation

There is no doubt that the shortage of resources is a considerable problem in health-care today. However, even if we were able to double resources, something which no political shift could achieve, there would certainly still be difficulties connected with making choices between the alternative claims on the central resource. Thus, the most efficient use of resources must be identified and chosen by a process of collecting information on the costs and benefits of alternative modes of care. As O'Donnell *et al.* (1988) have pointed out, there is very little evidence of the efficacy of alternative programmes and because of this choices are still made in ill considered ways. As far as community psychiatric nursing is concerned, there have been many claims that CPNs are cost effective (Illing *et al.*, 1990) but most of these claims are not based on any hard evidence. There are, at the time of writing, only three properly controlled studies of the efficacy of mental health nurses working in the community. The first of these, the widely quoted Paykel and Griffith study (1983), showed that CPNs were relatively cost effective in following up clients who had had psychiatric treatment. However, this study is now years out of date. In the second study, that of Marks (1985), a study of primary health care showed that nurse therapists trained on the ENB 650 course (Behavioural Psychotherapy) working with patients with phobic and obsessional disorders were cost beneficial both to the client and to the health care system. However, this focus of work is narrow and, as a recent study shows (Newell and Gournay, 1994), there are less than 100 nurse therapists (FTE) working in the UK today. In the third study, Gournay and Brooking (1992) showed that CPNs in primary health care working with patients with minor mental disorders were very expensive and, bearing in mind the possible much larger clinical gains achieved when working with people with serious mental illness, the economic data from this study indicated that there was little justification for CPNs continuing to work in primary health care with people with the less serious mental health problems.

Increasingly, all mental health professionals, including CPNs' will be asked to justify their work on grounds of economic efficiency and, therefore, community psychiatric nursing researchers will need to concentrate on economic as well as clinical outcomes in their evaluations of services. Again, this development will need community psychiatric nursing researchers to become acquainted with the principles of economic evaluation and, for some, this may be a taxing (no pun intended) exercise!

FUTURE RESEARCH METHODS

At the risk of repetition of some areas, it is worth describing some possible future priorities in research methodology.

More randomized controlled trials

As stated above, there has been a shortage of properly controlled evaluations of interventions in community psychiatric nursing research and this obviously needs to be addressed by the use of more randomized controlled trials. This is not to say that well-designed qualitative research should not be carried out but it is entirely possible to incorporate qualitative methodologies within the overall context of randomized controlled trials. Examples of such a strategy can be seen in the work of Paykel and Griffith (1983) and Gournay and Brooking (1992).

Greater use of the single case design

One great criticism of the nursing literature is the glut of case studies which are often used to justify particular approaches. Such case studies are often written without any thought apparently given to proper measures or any experimental control. Clinical psychology has long since used single cases as the basis of systematic enquiry and Hersen and Barlow (1976) have provided a number of excellent models of experiment. Such single case designs use multiple reliable measures of change and various experimental methods to dismantle experimental interventions such as multiple baseline and ABA (for an excellent account of such methods, see Barlow *et al.*, 1985). There is indeed an excellent case for saying that nursing journals (like many journals in psychology and psychiatry) should be reluctant to publish case studies without evidence that these studies use adequate measures of change and an appropriate single case methodology.

Greater use of 'psychological' methods

As indicated above, there is an extensive knowledge base in psychology relating to individual cognitive processes in various mental health problems and over treatment itself. For example, there are a whole host of measures of information processing, attribution, expectancy, perceived control and labelling (for an excellent review, see Brewin, 1988). Having said that, some researchers, for example Pollock (1986), have used measures such as the repertory grid to look at individual perceptions and it seems clear that future generations of community psychiatric nursing researchers need to be much more aware of the range of measures of cognition open to them and to develop discrimination regarding the appropriateness of each of these.

Increased use of appropriate statistical methods

Because of the very small number of mental health nurses and, indeed, nurses in general who have received training in research methods, there has been a reluctance to use statistical methods at any real level of sophistication on a widespread basis. If mental health nurses are really to vie for an equal footing with other health professionals, it will be very necessary for them to become more aware of the uses and, indeed, the limitations of more advanced statistical methods. There are several other influences which will increase pressure on mental health nurses to increase their expertise. First, funding bodies now require much more detailed accounts of proposed statistical analyses and certainly many of the Regional Health Authority research committees now require people applying for research grants to address key areas such as statistical power and effect size in their applications. The second influence is the increasing availability of various statistical packages and their widespread use on personal computers. It is now possible to carry out advanced statistical tests on fairly inexpensive machines and, therefore, there is no excuse for mental health nurses not using the appropriate statistical test. Third, journals are increasingly requiring more sophisticated statistical expertise from researchers and certainly the multidisciplinary journals will routinely require statistical tests which until recently were beyond the grasp of most mental health nursing researchers.

Having said that, there are dangers inherent in the increasing sophistication of statistical methods and, in particular, it may be that data derived from less than robust measures may be subjected to inappropriately complex statistical procedures. Indeed, in the author's view, it may be that there is an increasing use of complex methods such as analyses of covariance used on data which require much less than such methods, probably only requiring simple non-parametric tests!

CHANGES IN RESEARCH INFRASTRUCTURE

The first mental health nursing review for 25 years, commissioned by the Secretary of State, which is still being written at the time of writing this chapter, will undoubtedly say much about future changes in research infrastructure. The review findings will probably point to the necessity for adequate training for future generations of mental health nursing researchers and how the relatively small numbers of these people will need to work together in centres of excellence. There will obviously need to be proper resourcing of these centres and a corollary of this infrastructure development will be the need for establishing widely accessible information bases so that all mental health nurses can have access to research findings so that their practice may be appropriately informed. While mental health nursing research may change as a part of the more general changes in nursing research, there will also be developments in the ways in which research is funded (for example, the new Peckham Research Initiative) and future generations of mental health nurses may well find themselves operating in an arena with completely different rules and protocols.

CONCLUSION

Community psychiatric nursing research is a relatively new discipline and understandably there have been shortcomings in the quality of output. Nevertheless, there are a whole range of exciting possibilities for the future and providing that the present and future generation of community psychiatric nursing researchers integrate with other professionals in the mental health care field, there should be many positive outcomes which will result in higher levels of service provision for people with mental health problems. Nevertheless, it must be stressed that there is no cause for complacency, nor the self-congratulatory tones which occasionally emanate from gatherings of psychiatric nursing researchers. There is a need to look critically at the results of research output and at the present time there is no doubt that there is considerable scope for growth.

REFERENCES

Barlow, D.H., Hayes, S.C. and Nelson, R.O. (1985) *The Scientist Practitioner*, Pergamon, New York.

Bennett, J. (1991) Drugs and the CPN. *Nursing Times*, **44**, 38–40.

Birchwood, M. and Tarrier, N. (1992) *Innovations in the Psychological Management of Schizophrenia*, John Wiley and Sons, London.

Brewin, C.R. (1988) *Cognitive Foundations of Clinical Psychology*, LEA, London.

Brooker, C. (1990) *Community Psychiatric Nursing: A Research Perspective*, Chapman and Hall, London.

Brooker, C., Tarrier, N., Barrowclough, C., Butterworth, G. and Goldberg, D. (1992) Training community psychiatric nurses for psychological intervention. *British Journal of Psychiatry*, **160** 836–44.

Brooker, C. and White, E. (1993) *Community Psychiatric Nursing: A Research Perspective Vol. 2*, Chapman & Hall, London.

Brooking, J.I. (1986) *Psychiatric Nursing Research*, John Wiley and Sons, London.

Faugier, J. (1993) Human immunodeficiency virus (HIV) disease and drug misuse – research in issues for CPNs, *Community Psychiatric Nursing: A Research Perspective Vol. 2*, (eds C. Brooker and E. White), Chapman & Hall, London.

Foa, E. and Emmelkamp, P.M.G (1983) *Failures in Behaviour Therapy*, John Wiley and Sons, New York.

Gournay, K.J.M. (1991) The failure of exposure treatment in agoraphobia. *Journal of Advanced Nursing*, **6**, 1099–109.

Gournay, K.J.M. (1993) Trends in managing schizophrenia. *Nursing Standard*, 7(12), 31–7.

Gournay, K.J.M. and Brooking, J.I. (1992) *A Prospective Randomised Controlled Trial of the Efficacy of CPNs and GPs in Treating Patients with Minor Psychiatric Disorder in Primary Care*, Report to the Department of Health.

Gournay, K.J.M. and Brooking, J.I. (1993) Failure and dissatisfaction, *Community Psychiatric Nursing: A Research Perspective Vol. 2*, (eds C. Brooker and E. White), Chapman & Hall, London.

Gournay, K.J.M. and Brooking, J.I. (1994) The community psychiatric nurse in primary care: an outcome study. *British Journal of Psychiatry*, **165**, 231–8.

Hersen, M. and Barlow, D.H. (1976) *Single Case Experimental Designs: Strategies for Studying Behavior Change*, Pergamon, New York.

Illing, J., Drinkwater, C., Rogerson, T. *et al.* (1990) Evaluation of community psychiatric nurses in general practice, *Community Psychiatric Nursing: A Research Perspective*, (ed. C. Brooker), Chapman & Hall, London.

Marks, I.M. (1985) *Nurse Therapists in Primary Care*, RCN Publications, London.

Marks, I.M. (1987) *Fears, Phobias and Rituals*, Oxford Medical Publications, Oxford.

Newell, R. and Gournay, K.J.M. (1994) British nurses in behavioural psychotherapy: a 20 year follow-up. *Journal of Advanced Nursing*, **20**, 53–60.

O'Donnell, Maynard, A. and Wright, K. (1988) *The Economic Evaluation of Mental Health Care: A Review*, Centre for Health Economics, University of York.

Orem, D. (1985) *Nursing: Concepts of Practice*, McGraw-Hill, New York.

Paykel, E.S. and Griffith, J.H. (1983) *Community Psychiatric Nursing for Neurotic Patients*, RCN Publications, London.

Pollock, L.C. (1986) An introduction to the use of repertory grid technique as a research method and clinical tool for psychiatric nurses. *Journal of Advanced Nursing*, **11**, 439–45.

Roy, C. *(1976) Introduction to Nursing: An Adaption Model*, Prentice-Hall, Englewood Cliffs, New Jersey.

Roy, C. (1981) *Theory Construction in Nursing: An Adaption Model*, Appleton and Lange, New York.

Sarafino, E.P. (1990) *Health Psychology*, John Wiley and Sons, New York.

Sherman, P.S. and Porter, R. (1991) Mental health consumers as case manager aides. *Hospital and Community Psychiatry*, **42**(5), 494–8.

Stein, L. (1991) A systems approach to the treatment of people with chronic mental illness, *The Closure of Mental Hospitals*, (eds P. Hall and I.F. Brockington), Gaskell Royal College of Psychiatrists, London.

Thornicroft, G. (1994) The NHS and Community Care Act 1990. *Psychiatric Bulletin*, **18**(1), 13–17.

White, E. (1993) Community psychiatric nursing 1980 to 1990: a review of organisation, education and practice, in *Community Psychiatric Nursing: A Research Perspective Vol. 2*, (eds C. Brooker and E. White), Chapman & Hall, London.

CHAPTER 11

Implications and conclusions

Jerome Carson, Leonard Fagin and Susan Ritter

In this final chapter of the book each editor has written a separate contribution on an issue that particularly concerns them. Jerome Carson begins by discussing possible future directions for research into stress and coping in mental health nursing. Leonard Fagin examines the conflicting demands currently being made on community mental health nurses and suggests that being active members of multidisciplinary mental health teams may ease some of the pressures on them. In the final section Susan Ritter examines theories of nursing practice and links them to theories of stress. She highlights both the sheer complexity of the phenomenon we have labelled stress, as well as the diversity of people's responses to stress.

It is our sincere hope that this book will encourage others interested in the mental health nursing field to consider the effects that stress can have on workers and to consider creatively how the situation can be ameliorated. We hope that the material presented in this book will provide stimulation for other research workers.

To many research workers it is a sad but indisputable fact that research is seen by many clinicians as being a fairly meaningless academic activity which is of secondary importance to the real work, that of seeing patients. Even professions that pride themselves on having a strong research tradition in reality often have a poor research record (Pilgrim and Treacher, 1992). Workers with such a view of research will not therefore welcome my suggesting much more research into the issues of stress and coping in mental health nursing. However, I would like to suggest a number of issues that need to be addressed in future research studies. I begin, though, with a brief resumé of why this issue is so important.

The Claybury CPN Stress Study (presented in Chapters 5, 6, 7 and 8 of this book) has unequivocally demonstrated how psychiatric nursing can be a stressful profession. We found that not only are over 40% of CPNs suffering high stress as measured by Goldberg's General Health Questionnaire, but a similar percentage are also suffering high emotional burnout. Such findings should hopefully cause nurse managers to pause and ask two questions. Firstly, what is it that is causing CPNs so much stress and secondly what can we do to reduce stress levels in CPNs? The contributors to the present volume are not alone in being concerned about stress in mental health nursing. The Department of Health has recently identified the mental health of the NHS workforce as being a key priority area for research. While many of us no doubt have our own ideas on why mental health nurses might be so stressed, it is only through carefully conducted research studies that we will obtain objective answers to these questions. I would like to suggest the sorts of research studies that could provide us with such answers.

Perhaps the greatest omission from the current stress and coping literature is the absence of longitudinal studies. Almost all of the research conducted to date has been cross-sectional in nature (e.g. Power and Sharp, 1988). We now need to conduct studies that follow up mental health nurses over a number of years, to help us to appreciate how stress levels may alter over time. One might hypothesize, for example, that job transitions could be a particularly stressful time in the career of mental health nurses. If we were to study newly appointed staff nurses, we might predict that their stress level might be highest in the first six months post qualification and then possibly decline over time. Equally we might speculate that promotion, which not only brings extra money but also additional responsibility, might cause a further peak in stress levels.

Somewhat surprisingly, training to become a mental health professional might be even more stressful. Several studies (Cushway, 1992; Tobin and Carson, 1994) have demonstrated even higher stress levels in student groups. It would be illuminating to follow up a group of mental health nurses during their training and for the first three years after they qualify. Such a study would give us a much clearer picture of the developmental nature of stress and burnout in mental health professionals.

A second area meriting much greater attention is that of staff stress during the process of mental hospital closure. Nolan (1993) describes the historical development of mental health nursing and the key role of the asylums in the development of the profession. Claybury Hospital, the base for the CPN Stress Study, recently celebrated its centenary (Prior, 1993). Those of us who have worked in mental hospitals during the closure process will have been acutely aware of the effects this has had on both staff stress and morale.

In an earlier paper (Carson and Bartlett, 1990) we argued that many mental hospital nursing staff would find the transition to community care very difficult. Again one might intuitively predict that more recently qualified nursing staff would find the transition to community care less stressful. Somewhat surprisingly, this whole area has been massively under-researched. We are not therefore at present in a position to state exactly how mental hospital nurses cope with this, the most difficult of all transitions. To date the research effort has focused on the effects of reprovision on patients. The large TAPS (Team for the Assessment of Psychiatric Services) study of the closure of Friern and Claybury hospitals has concentrated almost exclusively on the effects of closure on patients (TAPS, 1988). Relatively few studies have looked at the effects of closure on staff (Ramon, 1992). While a number of mental hospitals remain open, I would argue that we desperately need to research the effects of the closure process on staff. Again this would require a longitudinal study.

A third area that merits further research attention is the study of organizational change within the health service. Reorganizations, which have always been a feature of the management of the health service, seem to have gained an increasing momentum in recent years, the purchaser–provider split and the establishment of health care trusts being only two in a long series of changes. Despite the apparent enthusiasm in both government and civil service circles for such draconian changes, we have little idea about their effect on staff. How will community mental health nurses be affected by the introduction of GP fundholding? How do all these changes affect staff on the ground? How do managers inform their staff of the changes? While managers are often at pains to reassure staff that they are the most important resource in the health service, treatment of staff does not often live up to the rhetoric. Together researchers and health service planners could monitor the effects of organizational changes on staff stress and morale levels. Unless staff feel cared for, they are unlikely to be able to give of their best to patients. Again one might hypothesize that senior and middle managers might be more affected by such changes than more junior staff. They are also responsible for implementing the changes.

A fourth area for future research in the field should be placing a greater emphasis on qualitative data. While we presented qualitative findings from the Claybury CPN Stress Study in Chapter 8, our main priority thus far has been to collect quantitative data. Such data often produce fascinating findings, but may not inform us why or how such findings may have come about. Witness our own finding that CPNs scoring high on our stress questionnaire have significantly more sick leave than CPNs scoring low. We assume that high stress levels are causing staff to take more time off sick. However, we know nothing of the pattern of staff sick leave. Again, we know that CPNs as a group take less sick leave than ward based colleagues, but we have not studied this issue in depth yet. What is needed is a more finegrained analysis at a local level to try and plot some of these associations. Qualitative methods have an invaluable role to play here. Handy (Chapter 4) has had CPNs use diaries to chart their workloads. Additionally researchers could 'shadow' CPNs to obtain a running narrative or commentary on how their clinical tasks affect their stress and coping abilities.

A fifth area for future research into stress would be to examine to what extent patients cause staff distress. In the Claybury CPN Stress Study, a number of CPNs reported being traumatized by suicide attempts. While a patient's suicide is probably one of the most traumatic events for many mental health professionals to deal with, working individually in the community the CPN is likely to perceive this as more stressful than when working as part of a ward team. Again dealing with violent incidents in ward settings (Wykes and Whittington, 1991) is going to be very different from handling the same episodes in the community. We need to ask the question, what characteristics of which types of patients cause staff most stress? Equally what strategies do staff need to employ to cope with or manage such incidents better?

Moving on to examine coping strategies, it would appear we have even more to learn here. While we used Professor Cooper's coping skill measure from his Occupational Stress Indicator, we also enquired about coping strategies in our Demographic Questionnaire and during our qualitative interviews. The most significant feature to emerge from the interviews and Demographic Questionnaire was the importance of social support from peers. The best way of coping with stress at work is to talk to a close colleague about it. The potential of social support as a stress intervention strategy has been examined by me in a study reported by Susan Ritter and colleagues in Chapter 9. Recently Judy Proudfoot, a PhD student at the Institute of Psychiatry, has compared social support group therapy (Carson, 1993) with cognitive therapy in a large cohort of unemployed people. The results of this work are not yet available, but should help us obtain a clearer picture of the role and utility of socal support as a coping strategy.

There are surprisingly few intervention studies with mental health nursing staff, though Nichols and Jenkinson (1991) provide a helpful manual for those thinking of running support groups for staff. The vast psychotherapy outcome literature should provide researchers with several models for evaluating effective stress intervention packages with nursing staff (Garfield and Bergin, 1986; Hersen *et al.*, 1984). There is a need to conduct a number of randomized control group trials looking at a range of interventions.

Undoubtedly, the best packages are likely to be eclectic in nature, encompassing a range of psychoeducational components (Wycherley, 1987). More common stress management techniques such as relaxation training and cognitive restructuring could be combined with time management, assertion skills, problem solving skills training and information on exercise and diet in a holistic approach. Such a holistic approach could then be evaluated with several groups of mental health nurses using a variety of methods: self-help manuals (a minimal intervention); three-day workshops; weekly sessions; fortnightly theme focused educational support groups.

The problem with such approaches, however, is that they tend to locate stress within the individual rather than seeing it as the product of a certain type of organizational environment. We need to be careful not to neglect interventions at an organizational level and to consider how effective intervening at this level would be, for instance, monitoring the effects of establishing a well-resourced new community mental health nursing team with good office facilities and secretarial back-up. Would stress and burnout levels be lower in a community team that was given adequate resources to fulfil its functions? It may even be the case that many of the psychological interventions we have developed for use with long-term client groups, such as social skills training (Carson and Holloway, 1994), may be more effective with staff groups.

Another research strategy would be to examine coping strategies in more depth. We could look at staff who cope well versus staff who cope poorly. What distinguishes these groups of staff? What can we learn from 'good copers' that we may be able to incorporate into stress intervention packages? Again, this would be best studied within a longitudinal design.

Jerome Carson

It is not unusual for mental health nurses to move into the community in order to escape the strict regimentation of the hospital and the imposition of consultant-led teams. CPNs value the extra freedom afforded to them by their jobs, their ability to structure their own time, opportunities to work with patients with a broad range of psychological disorders and the confirmation of their worth by general practitioners. It is therefore not surprising to find, at least initially in the career of a CPN, high levels of job satisfaction, but this is confined to actual work with patients. CPNs seem less satisfied by their new working

conditions and the increasing demands of large caseloads and conflicting sets of priorities.

Contract specifications under the health reforms of the 1990s
have imposed new restrictions and expectations, replacing the
old hospital hierarchies by primary care fundholding feudal organizations which also have the potential of placing CPNs in sub-
ordinate roles. The professional elders announced that unless CPNs
become more influential and organized, it is unlikely that they
will have much of a say on how mental health services should be
delivered and by whom (CPNA National Executive Council, 1994).
In this, they are equally positioned with other professional groups,
who have been replaced by fundholders and purchasing authorities as the main architects of the shape of the future in mental
health care. Although a great deal of lip service has been paid to the
involvement of users of mental health facilities, there is still little
evidence of this taking place at purchaser level and managerial and
political will, propped up by financial arguments, usually have the
final say.

In times when the professional voice is carrying less weight, where
the hollowness of 'consultation' is met with cynicism, where forests
of paperwork inundate and often replace time available for clinical
enterprise and where the culture of 'big brother' imposes defensive
professional manoeuvres aimed at securing the status quo and viability
of jobs, it is not surprising to find professionals who become dis-
affected, preferring to bury their heads in the sand in the hope that
it will all go away until it is time to retire or until catastrophe forces
sensible redirection. This attitude, all too prevalent in all health professionals working for the NHS in the 1990s, is indicative of resignation
and loss of vocational idealism and purposeful control. And this is
the fertile soil into which stress can extend its roots. Conversely, it
is surprising how much flack mental health workers will take if they
feel they are involved in services they can creatively influence and
direct, if they are breaking new ground, bringing new ideas and
energizing their working environment.

Stress becomes intolerable when you feel you are on your own.
We have found that although nurses appear to be using an average
or high number of coping skills, it did not necessarily follow that
the strategies employed were effective in reducing stress, but it
was clear that those CPNs who scored lower levels of stress gained
a great deal from the support they received from their peers, even
though adequate supervision from their managers and professional
elders was often absent or inadequate. But support should have a wider
base.

Multidisciplinary mental health community teams are difficult
organizations to manage and sustain (Watson, 1994) but they do

have the potential to offer a solid platform to all professionals who wish to participate equitably in the care of patients (Fagin, 1994). The moves CPNs made in the past decade towards primary care have often isolated nurses from other mental health professionals. It is uncommon in some services for nurses to do any joint work with colleagues from other disciplines and communications tend to be limited to occasional written missives. Certainly many opportunities are lost to learn from each other or to benefit from multiprofessional assessments. Whilst attachments to primary care have been progressive and necessary, they have been made at the expense of a broad outlook on mental health problems that include social, familial, biological and psychological perspectives. CPNs have been in danger of promoting themselves to primary care services as Jacks and Jills of all trades but masters of none, raising expectations which many find impossible to fulfil. This unilateral fragmentation of mental health services has stifled professional debate on how best to meet the variety of demands in locality based services. In promoting their own professional identity in this manner, CPNs have divorced themselves from an active participation in setting the direction of future mental health services.

It is time for CPNs to return to multidisciplinary teams equipped with their primary care experience and continuing to provide this active link with primary care levels. In doing this, CPNs would not only become a valuable asset to the community mental health team, they would also be inserting themselves into a necessary mutually supportive framework. This may not be universally popular with CPNs or with some general practitioners who have grown accustomed to having the near full attention of an accessible mental health worker on their premises. It will, however, offer the chance for CPNs to participate in a vision of care, rather than being reactive to immediate demands. It should also restore some equity of care to patients, avoiding two tier systems, by creating a common referral point to a team which could respond realistically to the level of need according to agreed priorities and resources available. This process can helpfully set boundaries for mental health professionals to work within. Stress is definitely heightened when you are unable to say no or when you are working without clear set criteria and limits.

These concepts are consistent with the implementation of *The Care Programme Approach* and the NHS and Community Care Act 1990 (Department of Health, 1990), whereby key workers will need to be identified for all patients discharged from hospital. CPNs will undoubtedly be selected as key workers in a substantial number of these discharges, forcing CPNs to work primarily with priority patients with enduring psychiatric illnesses. This is work that cannot be undertaken alone and requires firm support from the multidisciplinary team, with access to other professional advice and joint working. CPNs would be in an ideal position to bridge the communication gap between hospital and primary care services, because of their historic links with both these agencies. But I believe it goes further than this.

Professional developments for mental health nurses, and CPNs in particular, have the potential to bring the status of nurses into their rightful position within the mental health professional world. The introduction of Project 2000 (UKCC, 1986) and the ENB Framework and Higher Award (English National Board, 1990), by emphasizing nurses' academic background and degree qualifications, has endorsed the increasing confidence of their new roles, much on a par with university degrees of other professional groups. The expectation of further education under PREPP (Post-Registration Education and Practice Project) (UKCC, 1993) further enhances this position. Kevin Gournay in Chapter 10 emphasized the importance of CPNs becoming more active and thorough in carrying out research projects, especially if they are practice based.

All these endeavours should give heart to nurses re-entering multi-disciplinary practice as equals to other disciplines traditionally backed up by their higher training degrees, which in the past have created differential status within teams. Nurses need not fear that by joining multidisciplinary teams they will end up doing the 'dirty work' or reassuming the role of the 'doctor's handservant'. Their skills, if clearly defined and presented, can promote their sense of identity and professional autonomy, even when many of the clinical roles of care are shared. They will not only have a central clinical contribution to make to community mental health teams: they will also be in a position to lead them.

Progress will depend to a large extent on support offered to CPNs within their own management structures. It is often said that in most professions we are the architects of our own destinies. In that sense, we can also be our own worst enemies. Although managers often emanate from the professional groups they oversee, it is surprising how often they appear to shirk responsibilities for ensuring that their charges are not experiencing undue and unnecessary stress. In these situations staff experience their superiors as persecutory or as creating working conditions which perpetuate or enhance stress related conditions. Sometimes they are unaware of the first indications of staff under pressure or working on the verge of their capacities. In this context, it is not only important for staff to recognize indicators of stress and coping behaviours to handle it, but also for managers to learn to detect these conditions, especially when it is difficult for staff to communicate them out of a sense of loyalty or worries about job prospects. Adequate and empathic supervision, as well as staff groups, are often the barometers of staff tolerance and satisfaction.

The importance and relevance of the physical conditions in which staff work must not be underestimated. In our survey, CPNs regularly mentioned how the geography of the office prevented them from taking necessary respite, from having time to think or write their notes in peace and quiet. An efficient and adequately trained and supported secretary can be an inestimable asset to the team, especially if able to deal with anxious referrers until CPNs are ready to respond to them.

Flexibility of working arrangements is also a useful approach in preventing staff burnout. Part-time work, job sharing schemes, regular opportunities for diversification into special interests and training opportunities, as well as occasional paid sabbaticals, ensure staff loyalty and continuing healthy staff relationships. Unfortunately, the NHS is still many years behind its industrial counterparts in taking on board these measures to ensure continuing productivity.

The programme of hospital closures and community care arose out of decades of dissatisfaction with the dehumanizing aspects of institutionalization and the overwhelming stigmatization of patients with mental illnesses. This process has largely ignored two central facets of the translocation of services: the extra resources required to sustain people with mental illnesses in the community and the emotional and practical support required by carers, both professional and non-professional. The Claybury CPN Stress Study was set up to address this second issue. CPNs have been shown to experience high levels of stress in their current jobs and this surely cannot be ignored. Stress can blight promising careers, as well as substantially affect the level and quality of patient care. We are quite convinced that CPNs are not alone amongst mental health professionals in experiencing dissatisfaction and symptoms of stress. And yet, different professions are apprehensive about sharing these concerns or developing concerted actions to avoid burnout and resignation. It is time for all mental health professionals to join forces and ensure that their own needs, as well as those of their patients, clients or consumers, are adequately catered for.

Leonard Fagin

Regardless of the quality of available evidence, Rosen's (1959) observation remains pertinent: 'from the eighteenth century right down to the present day students of mental illness have been preoccupied' with the failure of society to create and maintain the conditions essential to the mental health of its members (p. 8). As this book shows, this failure is often conceptualized in terms of stress, sometimes with an implied suggestion that a sick individual is the product of a sick society, sometimes that the harmful sequelae of stress can be prevented by public or personal health measures or both.

Teachers of psychiatric and mental health nursing have supported the proposition that social forces have a pathoplastic effect on mental disorder by referring to the work of such writers as Mead (1934), Erikson (1950), Sullivan (1953), von Bertalanffy (1968) as mediated through the writing of Peplau (1952), Johnson (1980), Rogers (1976), King (1981), Neuman (1982), Roy (1976) and Sundeen *et al.* (1985). A wider assumption which underlies this proposition is that 'society' produces 'stresses' which lead to an inability to carry out activities of living whether at home or at work. At various times 'society' is represented by the family, the school, the workplace or the neighbourhood.

Often the inability to carry out activities of living is described as a form of 'illness' in the absence of a disease for which biochemical or radiological tests provide evidence. Menninger (1972) warns, 'Some afflictions are given diagnostic labels which are almost nicknames . . . a kind of jargon which does not attempt a precise diagnosis' (p. 40). Suppose that 'hypertension' is inferred from a reading of a person's blood pressure. Having an abnormal level of blood pressure is an affliction for which hypertension is a label. Stress is another label for a supposed affliction. Naming an affliction 'stress' sidesteps the difficulty of defining it but produces another difficulty in that a diagnostic label implies an illness/disease for which a suitable treatment can be selected.

Scadding (1967) discusses the point to which a given measure of blood pressure is labelled hypertension. The user of a criterion of the relationship between normality and abnormality names 'a specified common characteristic or set of characteristics' (Scadding, 1967) which represent deviation from the norm and so makes a diagnosis. This means that an individual can be thought of as being ill, while having no disease. Conversely the diagnosis of disease is 'a necessary, but by no means sufficient basis for clinical decision' (Cawley, 1983, p. 781), as in the case of a person whose brain scan shows a cyst to which his psychotic symptoms and behaviour cannot be attributed. These considerations require the clinician to assemble his or her data scrupulously and attend to the many factors influencing a person's presentation of 'illness'. They imply that health and illness, far from being on a continuum, are complex and overlapping concepts which are themselves complex groupings of factors.

If a diagnostic label is applied on the basis of a sample of available data it is likely that powerful influences are missed – influences which are also likely to confound attempts to intervene. A reading of a person's blood pressure occurs in the context of that individual's history, present circumstances and heredity. The blood pressure becomes less a sign or a symptom and more a sampling of one aspect of an individual at a specific moment. What is inferred from this sample depends on what the clinician is prepared to take into account. It follows that 'a given disease can produce different "illnesses" in different people' (Cawley, 1983, p. 772), while 'diseases keep disappearing but sickness remains' (Menninger, 1972, p. 37).

Cawley suggests that because 'illness' is the product of the unique interaction between an individual's context, heredity and history (as well as the clinician's diagnostic 'culture'), it must be scrupulously defined by the clinician in partnership with that individual. This is termed an idiographic approach – one that attends to the facets of the individual that are as personal as his or her signature or thumbprint. However, a number of influential nursing writers, such as those listed above, attempt to describe individual 'clients', 'persons', 'patients', 'patiency' or 'unitary man' in a rhetoric which includes terms like health, wellness, balance, disharmony, adjustment and responsibility. This purports to be an idiographic approach. It is rather a nomothetic approach – one that states a set of laws. In the course of their writing they have tried to appropriate a remarkable range of territory as being suitable for nursing intervention. These descriptions of nursing care objectify the extremely complex and fluid issues outlined above. They claim more for nursing than is justified by the evidence they present. They are misapplications of biological research. And they illuminate some of the difficulties experienced by psychiatric and mental health nurses in the course of their work.

Using a military analogy Neuman (1982) asserts that stressors are phenomena which penetrate lines of defence. Instability results from this invasion. The goals of nursing care are to identify stressors at Caplan's (1961) three levels of prevention (primary, secondary, tertiary) and to intervene by treating symptoms as they occur in clients' coping patterns, expectations and motivation. The 'illness', so far as it can be inferred from this description, is a failure to adapt to environmental circumstances. Sundeen *et al.* (1985) do not rely on a notion of equilibrium but rather a health–illness continuum where health and wellness coincide. But they do use Caplan's (1961) levels of prevention mixed with a variety of other material to suggest that the nurse's task is to help 'people with health problems' (p. 156) move to 'higher' levels of wellness.

Like Neuman (1982), Johnson (1980) defines health in terms of stability or 'system balance' which is destabilized by internal or environmental changes. The goals of nursing include restoration of stability by imposing external regulatory or control mechanisms, changing 'structural units in desirable directions' (Johnson, 1980).

King (1981) argues that the 'dynamic life experience of a human being implies continuous adjustment to stressors in the internal and external environment through continuous use of one's resources to achieve maximum potential for daily living' (p. 5). Like Neuman and Johnson, King refers to system balance as being synonymous with 'health', but she is more explicit about the nature of the 'illness' which is, she says, 'A deviation from normal . . . an imbalance in a person's biological structure or in his psychological makeup, or in a conflict in a person's social relationships' (p. 3). In King's terms, therefore, disease is only one kind of illness. Like Neuman and Johnson, she describes nursing care as having the goal of helping 'recipients of care' (p. 8) to adjust to changes in their daily activities.

Orem (1980) also defines health as a system in balance, by which she appears to mean a system that is functional and integrated with motivation and the ability to take care of itself. Among self-care needs, Orem includes the need to be normal and the prevention of hazards to life and well-being. By defining ill health in terms of a range of inability to take care of oneself, Orem has an easier task of defining nursing care as partly or entirely acting on behalf of a person in order to supply deficits in self-care.

Peplau (1952) provides a simple definition of 'illness' as interference to the normal course of life activities. Roy (1976), in contrast, provides the following definitions: 'The person adapting in health and illness is the patiency of nursing care' (p. 184) and 'the patiency of nursing [is] the person as an adaptive system receiving stimuli from the environment which are inside and outside his zone of adaptation' (p. 184). The recipient of nursing care is a person who is ill or is potentially ill or is adapting to his or her environment.

Rogers (1980) warns that the principles that she sets out in her introduction to the theoretical basis of nursing (Rogers, 1976) 'have validity only within the context of the conceptual system of unitary man' (p. 333). The term 'introduction' belies the scope that Rogers (1976) claims for nursing intervention, ranging from telepathic communication to therapeutic touch. She rejects terms like disease and pathology in favour of terms like undesirable errors in the human field (Rogers, 1980). The work of the nurse is to facilitate clients in moving towards a state of greater well-being.

Given such a wide scope for nursing action the individual nurse is faced with the responsibility of attempting to 'assess' every facet of a person's life, not primarily in order to help that person make sense of his or her predicament but in order to legitimize a wide range of interventions whose rationale is 'adjustment' or 'adaptation'.

Three consequences ensue. Firstly such a diffuse and global remit invites failure by the person who attempts to accomplish it. This failure is likely to lead to internal self-criticism as well as criticism from outside. The disparity between personal expectation and personal achievement may be reflected in organizational conflict.

Secondly the nurse becomes an object of speculation about his or her system balance. Evidence of imbalance may be taken as evidence of an 'illness'. To have an illness is to require treatment. Not to accept treatment is evidence of deficient 'motivation' which in turn is further evidence of system imbalance. To comply with treatment is termed taking responsibility. Failure to take responsibility for oneself is also evidence of system imbalance. The impossibility of achieving personal or organizational goals becomes an affliction which may be labelled stress. It is a short step to attributing the causes of stress to internal qualities of the person.

Global assertion of nursing responsibility for any perceived 'system imbalance' combined with an inability to fulfil more than a limited aspect of that responsibility suggests why morale among nurses is fragile. When low morale is understood as a symptom of personal 'deficit' or 'deviation from the normal' (Orem, 1980; King, 1981), it renders the individual's fitness for his her work subject to scrutiny. In such circumstances it is not surprising that nurses may be reluctant to seek help and why they are likely to adopt exaggerated versions of what Menninger (1972) calls the minor emergency mechanisms of everyday life: tea, coffee, cigarettes and alcohol.

Thirdly, these nursing writers account for stress, its consequences and possible nursing interventions in ways that obscure the accounts of stress in the literature. When Selye's theory of the general adaptation syndrome was first published in Britain in 1936 it was disregarded. But after cortisone was synthesized in the mid 1940s and used to treat rheumatoid arthritis in Italy and the USA, Selye's account of the ways in which the human organism responds to internal as well as external 'attack' was made the centrepiece of a European meeting on rheumatic disease (Selye, 1936; Leader, 1950). While on the one hand the influence of Selye's general theory is by now incalculable, on the other hand, advances in neuroendocrinology and the identification of neuropeptides and transmitters whose function is still to be determined mean that the nature of adaptation is even more complex than Selye proposed.

Put at its simplest, the infinite personal characteristics and circumstances which make response to stress unpredictable are another reason for attending to Cawley's position as stated above. 'Illness or 'stress' must be scrupulously defined in terms of the personal facets of the individual in relation to his or her surroundings.

Because psychiatric and mental health nursing theory contains few operational (empirically testable) definitions and fewer tests of validity, appraisal of the research into the effects of stress on psychiatric and mental health nurses necessarily rests more on the stress literature than on the nursing literature. This is not a desirable procedure because the results of any given study will be affected not only by the idiographic features of individual nurses in relation to their environment, but by the intangible and measured characteristics of psychiatric and mental health nursing practice. A further confounding problem is that studies of stress in psychiatric and mental health nursing do not share assumptions or vocabulary, making comparison and replication difficult.

Susan Ritter

REFERENCES

Caplan, G. (1961) *An Approach to Community Mental Health*, Tavistock, London.

Carson, J. (1993) Manual for Social Support Group Therapy, unpublished manuscript, Institute of Psychiatry, London.

Carson, J. and Bartlett, H. (1990) *Care in the Community. Are the Staff as Stressed by the Changes as the Patients?* Paper given at TAPS Annual Conference, St Bartholomews Hospital, London.

Carson, J. and Holloway, F. (1994) Interventions with long term clients, in *Collaborative Community Mental Health Care*, (eds M. Watkins, N. Hervey, S. Ritter and J. Carson), Edward Arnold, London.

Cawley, R. (1983) Psychiatric diagnosis: what we need. *Psychiatric Annals*, **13**(10), 772–82.

CPNA National Executive Council (1994) Negotiating contracts for CPN teams. *Mental Health Nursing*, **14**(2), 22.

Cushway, D. (1992) Stress in clinical psychology trainees. *British Journal of Clinical Psychology*, **31**, 169–79.

Department of Health (1990) *The Care Programme Approach*, Circular HC90 (23), HMSO, London.

English National Board (1990) *Framework for Continuing Education and Training for Nurses, Midwives and Health Visitors*, Project Paper 3, ENB, London.

Erikson, E. (1950) Childhood and Society, W.W. Norton, New York.

Fagin, L. (1994) Teamwork among professionals involved with disturbed families, *Collaborative Community Mental Health Care*, (eds M. Watkins, N. Hervey, S. Ritter and J. Carson), Edward Arnold, London.

Garfield, S. and Bergin, A. (eds) (1986) *Handbook of Psychotherapy and Behaviour Change*, John Wiley and Sons, New York.

Hersen, M., Michelson, L. and Bellack, A. (eds) (1984) *Issues in Psychotherapy Research*, Plenum, New York.

Johnson, D. (1980) The behavioural systems model for nursing, *Conceptual*

Models for Nursing Practice, (eds J. Riehl and C. Roy, Appleton Century Crofts, Norwalk, CT.

King, I. (1981) *A Theory for Nursing*, John Wiley and Sons, New York.

Leader, J. (1950) The general adaptation syndrome. *British Medical Journal*, 1, 1410–11.

Mead, G. (1934) *Mind, Self and Society*, University of Chicago Press, Illinois.

Menninger, K. (1972) *The Vital Balance*, Viking, New York.

Neuman, B. (ed.) (1982) *The Neuman Systems Model: Applications to Nursing Education and Practice*, Appleton Century Crofts, New York.

Nichols, K. and Jenkinson, J. (1991) *Leading a Support Group*, Chapman & Hall, London.

Nolan, P. (1993) *A History of Mental Health Nursing*, Chapman & Hall, London.

Orem, D. (1980) *Nursing: Concepts of Practice*, McGraw Hill, New York.

Peplau, H. (1952) *'Interpersonal Relations in Nursing*, G.P. Putnams, New York.

Pilgrim, D. and Treacher, A. (1992) *Clinical Psychology Observed*, Routledge, London.

Power, K. and Sharp, G. (1988) A comparison of sources of nursing stress and job satisfaction among mental handicap and hospice nursing staff. *Journal of Advanced Nursing*, 13, 726–32.

Prior, E. (1993) *Claybury – A Century of Caring*, Forest Healthcare Trust, London.

Ramon, S. (1992) The persective of professional workers: living with ambiguity, ambivalence and challenge, in *Psychiatric Hospital Closure – Myths and Realities*, (ed. S. Ramon), Chapman & Hall, London.

Rogers, M. (1976) *Introduction to the Theoretical Basis of Nursing*, F. Davis, Philadelphia.

Rogers, M. (1980) Nursing: a science of unitary man, in *Conceptual Models for Nusing Practice*, (eds J. Riel and C. Roy), Appleton Century Crofts, Norwalk, CT.

Rosen, G. (1959) Social stress and mental disease from the eighteenth century to the present: some origins of social psychiatry. *Millbank Memorial Fund Quarterly*, 37, 5–32.

Roy, C. (1976) *Introduction to Nursing*, Prentice-Hall, Englewood Cliffs, NJ.

Scadding, J. (1967) Diagnosis: the clinician and the computer. *Lancet*, 2, 877–82.

Selye, H. (1936) Thymus and adrenals in the response of the organism to injuries and intoxications. *British Journal of Experimental Pathology*, 17, 234–48.

Sullivan, H. (1953) *The Interpersonal Theory of Psychiatry*, W.W. Norton, New York.

Sundeen, S., Stuart, G., Rankin, E. and Cohen, S. (1985) *Nurse–client Interaction*, C.V. Mosby, St. Louis.

Team for the Assessment of Psychiatric Services (1988) *Preliminary Report on Baseline Data from Friern and Claybury Hospitals*, NETRHA, London.

Tobin, J. and Carson, J. (1944) Stress and the student social worker. *Social Work and Social Sciences Review* (in press).

United Kingdom Central Council (1986) *Project 2000: A New Preparation for Practice*, UKCC, London.

United Kingdom Central Council (1993) *Post-registration and Practice Project*, UKCC Register, 12, 10.

Von Bertalanffy, L. (1968) *General Systems Theory*, George Braziller, New York.

Watson, G. (1994) Multidisciplinary working and co-operation in community care. *Mental Health Nursing*, **14**(2), 18–21.
Wycherley, B. (1987) *The Living Skills Pack*, SETRHA, Bexhill.
Wykes, T. and Whittington, R. (1991) Coping strategies used by staff following assault by a patient: an exploratory study. *Work and Stress*, **5**(1), 37–48.

Index

Page numbers appearing in **bold** refer to figures and page numbers appearing in *italics* refer to tables.